Voluntary Assisted Dying

An International Perspective on End of Life Choices for Cancer Patients

Voluntary Assisted Dying
An International Perspective on End of Life Choices for Cancer Patients

Ruth E Board and Peter Selby

EBN HEALTH

OXFORD, UK

EBN Health
An imprint of Evidence-based Networks Ltd
85 Newland, Witney,
Oxfordshire OX28 3JW, UK

Tel: +44 1865 522326
Email: info@ebnhealth.com

Web: www.ebnhealth.com

Distributed worldwide by:
Ingram Content Group
Ingramcontent.com

ISBN Print   978 173942 702 3
ISBN ebook   978 173942 703 0

Series design by Thomson Digital, Noida, India
Typeset by Thomson Digital, Noida, India

Contents

Contributors

This book is a descriptive review. It updates and extends our previous book "End of Life Choices for Cancer Patients. An International Perspective" published by EBN Health in 2020. RB, DE and PS initiated the book; RB and PS took oversight and edited the whole book.

We searched the NLM-NCBI PubMed dataset from 2020 to the time of writing for each chapter, and PS reviewed all titles and selected abstracts and full papers to read and include where they presented new information and data of general relevance to AD. He also searched online for formal reports from official sources on Assisted Dying development and delivery from the international jurisdictions that permit Assisted Dying. We have given priority to systematic and scoping reviews, which reduces the risk of publication bias, and to formal reports, where they are available. In general, we gave a lower priority to opinion pieces and press reports except where they gave insights into the public debate.

RB and PS coauthored chapters 1-9 and 11; IB provided valuable feedback on chapter 2; RB, PS, SK, AS and EA coauthored Chapter 3; AS authored chapter 10; PS, RB, and DE authored Chapter 12.

Professor Ruth E. Board (RB), Consultant in Medical Oncology, Lancashire Teaching Hospitals NHS Trust, Preston UK; Honorary Clinical Professor, University of Central Lancashire.

Dr Suzanne Kite (SK), Consultant/Lead Clinician Palliative Care, The Leeds Teaching Hospitals NHS Trust, President, Association for Palliative Medicine

Mr Abeezar Sarela PhD (AS) Consultant in Upper GI & Bariatric Surgery, St. James's University Hospital, Hon. Senior Lecturer in Surgery, University of Leeds School of Medicine

Dr Elspeth Aspinall (EA) GP, Joint Strategic Lead for Grampian Palliative Care MCN, Joint Lead Grampian Primary Care Cancer, Clinical Lead Frailty, Cancer and Palliative Care Aberdeenshire HSCP

Dr Isra Black (IB), Associate Professor, Vice Dean (International), UCL Faculty of Laws, University College London

Duncan Enright (DE), Managing Director, EBN Health

Professor Peter Selby (PS), Emeritus Professor of Cancer Medicine, University of Leeds, Leeds, UK; Visiting Professor, University of Lincoln, UK and Past President, Association of Cancer Physicians

Acknowledgements

The editors and authors are grateful to all of their colleagues, clients and patients who have inspired them to prepare this book and to seek to improve the choices available for cancer patients. The authors, editors and contributors would like to thank the participants of the workshop in Leeds in 2019, and the subsequent book published in 2020 for their contribution to the discussion on this important topic which guided this update.

The editors and authors warmly acknowledge the support they have received in preparing this book. Nicole Goldman conducted the extensive searches, coordinated and oversaw the book's final drafts. The editors, authors and the publisher are most grateful to the Association of Cancer Physicians for their support and advice during the development of this book. We are very grateful to all staff at EBN Health for their expert work, support, goodwill and interest in our purpose in preparing the book.

All of the authors and contributors would like to thank their employers and honorary employers for their support and for encouraging them to contribute to healthcare education, training, and research. The views expressed in this work are personal and do not reflect views or positions held by their employers.

Association of Cancer Physicians Problem Solving series

The 'Problem Solving' series of cancer-related books are developed and prepared by the Association of Cancer Physicians (ACP), often in partnership with one or more other specialist medical organisations. As the representative body for medical oncologists in the UK, the ACP has a broad set of aims, including education for our own members and for non-members, including interested clinicians, healthcare professionals and the public.

The ACP has set out to supplement regular and essential professional training and continuing education with workshops and publications that address important developments which will influence oncology and patient well-being. These occur approximately annually. The Problem-Solving series is a planned sequence of publications that derive from this programme initiated in 2014 with Problem Solving in Acute Oncology followed by Problem Solving in Older Cancer Patients in 2016, Problem Solving through Precision Oncology in 2017, Problem Solving in Patient-Centred and Integrated Cancer Care in 2018 and Problem Solving in Immunotherapy in 2019. Problem Solving in Acute Oncology 2nd Edition and also End of Life Choices for Cancer Patients were published in 2020 and Cancer and Fertility in 2021.Problem Solving in Interventional Oncology was published in 2023.

The publication involves considerable work from members and other contributors, and this work is done without remuneration as an educational service. We have been delighted with the standard of the publications, and they have been well received. The BMA prize for Best Oncology Book of the Year was awarded to Problem Solving in Older Cancer Patients in 2016, Problem Solving in Precision Oncology in 2017 and Problem Solving in Patient-Centred and Integrated Cancer Care in 2018.

In the present publication, the important and controversial topic of Voluntary Assisted Dying is addressed for the second time to reflect the rapidly changing landscape globally and recent parliamentary bills in the British Isles.

The ACP wishes to thank all of the contributors to this book, our previous publications and those which are yet to come.

Andrew Wardley, Chairman, Association of Cancer Physicians, Peter Selby, Past President, Association of Cancer Physicians and Helena Earl, President, Association of Cancer Physicians

Preface

End of Life Choices for Cancer Patients. An Updated International Perspective 2025

There have been impressive improvements in the diagnosis and treatment of cancer in recent decades. In economically advantaged countries with well-developed healthcare systems, over 50% of all cancer patients achieve long-term survival and are probably cured. Not only has survival improved radically for cancer patients but also there has been an increasing focus on the quality of patients' lives, on improving the patient experience of care and on developing effective support for the very many cancer survivors.

Despite the progress in cancer treatment, unfortunately a substantial number of cancer patients will still ultimately die of their disease. For many this will follow periods of successful treatment which resulted in good remissions and good quality of life. Helping patients to make the right choices about their care towards the end of their lives is one of the greatest and most challenging responsibilities of all healthcare professionals.

Legal change on the provision of assisted dying by healthcare professionals has occurred in a substantial number of jurisdictions. Legislation to permit assisted dying based on intolerable suffering is in place in Canada, Spain, Portugal, Luxembourg, Belgium, the Netherlands, Austria, and Switzerland. Legislation to permit assisted dying based on established terminal illness is in place in in the United States (Washington, Oregon, Hawaii, California, Colorado, New Mexico, Maine, Vermont, New Jersey and the District of Columbia), Australia (South Australia, Western Australia, Queensland, Victoria, Tasmania, NSW) and in New Zealand. There is partially permissive legislation in Columbia, Montana, Germany and Italy. The House of Commons in Westminster has voted to support a Bill to legalise Voluntary Assisted Dying which will now proceed to the House of Lords. Parliaments in Scotland, Jersey and the Isle of Man have also voted in favour of Bills to legalise Voluntary Assisted Dying.

In 2020, we published our first book on the topic. In the light of current proposed changes in the law, we now bring the book up to date to 2025.

Our intention in this work is:

- To provide updated information to support healthcare professionals and the public in the further consideration of the issues surrounding Voluntary Assisted Dying.
- To provide updated information to support the scrutiny and development of legislation to ensure the effective development and delivery of appropriate healthcare services and the appropriate protection of patients.
- To provide a resource to assist patient and professional groups who may be involved in education, training and professional development and who wish to update their knowledge of this area.

Chapter 1: Introduction, Public Opinion and the Social Context of Death

There have been impressive improvements in the diagnosis and treatment of cancer in recent decades. In economically advantaged countries with well-developed healthcare systems, over 50% of all cancer patients achieve long-term survival and are probably cured. This much-improved outcome may be compared with a figure of only about 25% in the latter half of the 20th century in these countries. Not only has survival improved radically for cancer patients but also there has been an increasing focus on the quality of patients' lives, on improving the patient-experience of care and on developing effective support for the very many cancer survivors.[1]

Major scientific and technological developments are continuing, and the practice of oncology is becoming more precise, and with more accurate patient selection for appropriate treatment. In addition to surgery, radiotherapy and systemic therapies, there are important developing and successful new modalities of treatment, including vaccine and cellular therapies and interventions that can destroy tumours using heat, cold, electricity, radio waves and ultrasound, without major surgical procedures. There still remain many challenges to be addressed if we are to continue to improve cancer therapy and its outcome. Not only must we vigorously pursue the scientific and technical advances that are providing improvements, but we must also ensure that care for cancer patients is well organised, with timely access to the appropriate diagnostic tests and treatments. We must provide high-quality and timely support for patients who have acute medical problems and complications from cancer. We must recognise that cancer is most commonly a disease of elderly people and adjust our approaches to make them feasible and acceptable for all patients.[1–8]

Despite the progress outlined above, a substantial number of cancer patients will still ultimately die of their disease. For many, this will follow periods of successful treatment that resulted in good remissions and good quality of life. However, when patients relapse, the disease may become resistant to available treatment. Helping patients to make the right choices about their care towards the end of their lives is one of the greatest and most challenging responsibilities of all healthcare professionals. Choosing treatments to relieve symptoms is often difficult. Decisions on the continuation of specific anticancer treatments to prolong life or relieve symptoms are complex and uncertain and depend greatly on our ability to elicit the patient's needs and preferences. The involvement of partners, family and friends is often important but must be achieved without overshadowing the patient's own views. Oncology and palliative care professionals from many disciplines work together in teams in order to provide the best possible help for their patients.

A workshop "End of life choices for cancer patients: an international perspective" was held in Leeds in May 2019 and brought together colleagues from oncology disciplines, palliative care, law, nursing and professions allied to medicine. The goals were to allow an exchange of information through formal presentations and discussion:

- to better inform the wider community about developments in choices in end-of-life care for cancer patients in the UK and internationally;
- to be better able to answer questions from patients and respond to their requests;
- to have a balanced and well-informed dialogue about choices available to patients;
- to provide a basis of information for future educational activities.

The workshop was the basis of a short book "End of Life Choices for Cancer Patients. An International Perspective" published by EBN in 2020.[1]

There was a consensus in the workshop that the decisions about changing legislation should be influenced most by social, legal and political opinion and should not be heavily influenced by those of healthcare professionals. The views of healthcare professionals are important, not because they should guide or shape public opinion but because these professionals are closely involved in the provision of good-quality care for patients at the end of life and will continue to be so. Any legislative change will have a very substantial impact on the patterns and quality of clinical practice and communication with patients.

In 2024 and 2025, the UK Parliament considered a Bill to legalise Assisted Dying (AD) under rigorous conditions. It was passed by the House of Commons and is proceeding to the House of Lords in the process of further scrutiny and developing the legislation.[9] Its impact has been studied in support of the consideration of the legislation.[10]

This publication updates the 2020 book. Our multiprofessional team of authors intends to provide updated information to support our professional colleagues, other professionals, legislators, and the public in the further consideration of appropriate legislation and if it is passed into law, its implementation.

Definitions

The topic of AD involves a wide range of terms and definitions that are constantly changing. In the workshop and publications, we have used the terminologies shown in Box 1.1.

Box 1.1 Definitions.

- Assisted Dying: (Voluntary) includes euthanasia and assisted suicide.
- Euthanasia: An intervention undertaken with the intention of ending a life to relieve suffering.

Some common (and often confusing) modifiers of euthanasia are:
  - Active: A deliberate intervention to end life.
  - Passive: Withdrawal/withholding of life-sustaining treatment.
  - Voluntary: At the request of the person killed.
  - Involuntary: In the absence of a request by the person killed, although that person is competent. – Non-voluntary: In the absence of a request by the person killed, when that person is not competent and has not made an advance request for euthanasia.

- Assisted suicide: Any act that intentionally helps another person to commit suicide, for example by providing him or her with the means to do so. In the Netherlands, assisted suicide is often included in the term euthanasia. Legal regimes often permit only physician-assisted suicide.
- Physician-assisted death: This includes physician-administered voluntary euthanasia and physician-assisted suicide.
- Medical assistance in dying (MAID): Used most recently in Canada and includes physician-assisted suicide and clinician-administered voluntary euthanasia.

Current public opinion

The British Social Attitudes Survey (BSA) is a well-respected source of information on public opinion, generally regarded as using robust methodology with good sample sizes. Between 1983 and 2016, the BSA asked the British public the question "Should the law allow a doctor to end the life of a patient with painful incurable disease?" The responses were notably stable with 75–82% of respondents answering "Yes".[11]

In 2017, the BSA asked in greater detail looking at several scenarios with responses in five categories including "definite" or "probable" support for AD, which the BSA refers to as voluntary euthanasia and which can be found at.[12]

They asked, "Should the law allow voluntary euthanasia in this situation?". The %age of "definite" and "probable" positive answers is given in brackets after each scenario.

By a doctor for someone with an incurable and painful illness from which they will die (79%)
By a close relative for someone with an incurable and painful illness from which they will die (39%)
By a doctor for someone with an incurable and painful illness from which they will not die (50%)
By a doctor for someone who is dependent, but not in pain or danger of death (50%)

To evaluate current opinion on the change in legislation to permit AD in England and Wales, the King's College London Policy Institute and Complex Life and Death Decisions Group conducted a nationally representative survey of over 2000 adults in England and Wales on the issues that relate to AD in 2024.[13] The main findings were:

- Two-thirds of the public back the legislation of AD within this parliament.
- The public have concerns about the risks of AD even when they are broadly supportive of its legislation.
- Supporters of AD prioritise pain relief and dignity, while opponents worry most about risks to the vulnerable.
- Most of the public want AD to be available on the NHS although they are uncertain about the financial impact of legislation on the NHS.
- Patients with mental health conditions are perceived to be most at risk of potential misuse of legal AD.
- Age and ethnicity are key dividing lines in public opinion on AD, with younger people being notably less likely to back AD than older people. People from minority ethnic groups are less likely than white people to support AD legislation.

YouGov conducted polls on the topic of Assisted Dying in November 2024 and May 2025, during a period of intense debate across the UK. They reported that 75% of Britons support assisted dying in principle, with little change over this timeframe, and similar support to that recorded in previous decades. Most Britons supported assisted dying in both principle and practice and 73% supported the current Assisted Dying Bill with 35% strongly supporting it and 38% somewhat supporting it in its present form.[14,15]

Opinium UK,[16] sponsored by the campaign group Dignity in Dying, which is a supporter of legislation to permit AD, conducted an online survey amongst a sample of 10,897 UK Adults in February 2024,[17] (which includes a link to the Excel Spreadsheet). Their sample size allows comments on diversity of the responses across the country and in different communities. To the question *"To what extent would you support making it legal to seek "assisted dying" in the UK?"* they categorised responses to be "Strongly Supportive" or "Somewhat Supportive" as "Net Support" and similar categories for opposition as "Net Oppose". Net Support was recorded for 75%

of all respondents and Net Oppose for 14% with 11% "Don't Know". The Net Support result was consistent (over 70%) across the UK Devolved Nations and English regions except London (67%) and Northern Ireland (66%). Other groups whose Net Support scores were below 70% were those declaring themselves to be Religious (66%); all Christians (69%); Catholic (65%); Muslims (34%); Hindu (58%); Jewish (61%); Sikh (62%); Asian people (48%); Black people (47%) and those aged 18–24 years (68%).

People reporting themselves to be Disabled recorded Net Support at 78%. NHS employees recorded 79% Net Support.

Ipsos conducted an AD poll in July 2023[18] in 1128 Online British adults aged 16–75. The information below was given to respondents before they answered the questions in this survey.

"The next few questions are about assisted dying in the UK. Assisted dying refers to a patient aged 18 or over being provided with life-ending medication if at least two doctors think that all the following conditions were met:

- *The patient would need to be of sound mind,*
- *The patient would be terminally ill and it is believed that they have 6 months or less to live,*
- *The patient would have made a voluntary, clear and settled decision to end their life (and made and signed a declaration to that effect in the presence of a witness), with time to consider all other options,*
- *The patient has been resident in the country for at least a year,*
- *The High Court confirms it is satisfied that these conditions have been met,*
- *If the conditions are met, a health professional may help to prepare and assist with the medication, but the decision to self-administer the medicine and the final act of doing so must be taken by the patient themselves. Assisted dying is not currently legal in the UK".*

Their questions and the response rates reported included:
"Should it be legal for a doctor to assist a terminally ill patient in ending their life by prescribing life ending medication?
Yes 65% No 17%
Should it be legal for a doctor to assist a terminally ill patient in ending their life by administering life ending medication?
Yes 61% No 21%
Do you think that it should be legal or not for a doctor to assist a patient (aged 18 or over in ending their life, if they are not terminally ill, but are physically suffering in a way that the patient finds unbearable and which cannot be cured or improved with existing medical science, and where the patient has expressed a clear desire to end their life? Assume that the other conditions for assisted dying outlined above are met.
Yes 55% No 22%
And do you think it should be legal or not for a doctor to assist a patient aged 18 or over in ending their life, if they are not terminally ill, but are mentally or emotionally suffering in a way that the patient finds unbearable and which cannot be cured or improved with existing medical science, and where the patient has expressed a clear desire to end their life? Assume that the other conditions for assisted dying outlined above are met. Yes 36% No 40%"

The complexity and importance of cultural and religious views[19] and the concerns and opinions of disabled and disadvantaged people are addressed in Chapter 8.

Overall, and over a long period there does appear to be a settled view in the UK public that they support AD under carefully regulated conditions, even when those conditions are clearly expressed in the questions posed. Support for AD for terminal illness is stronger than that for people with intolerable suffering who do not have a terminal diagnosis for which a period of life expectancy is defined. There are important groups within the UK who do not support this majority view, and whose views are discussed in Chapter 8.

The social context and the Lancet Commission on the Value of Death

Since our publication in 2020,[1] there have been several publications on the wider issues surrounding the social context of death, notably the "Lancet Commission on the Value of Death: bringing death back into life" in 2022[20] and a meta-systematic review on the conditions of a good death in 2021.[21] While the many and complex global issues which were highlighted are beyond the scope of our publication, the authors believe that discussions and decisions on the topic of AD, should be set in this wider context.

The Lancet Commission takes a global view of the issues surrounding death in the 21st century,[20] bringing out that in much of the world, inadequate healthcare means that many people are dying of preventable or readily treatable conditions without access to basic symptom control. On the other hand, in economically advantaged countries, many people may die in hospital while receiving treatment which carries very little chance of cure or long-term improvement, but with a trend towards marginalisation of the role of their families and communities. The authors note that "relationships and networks are being replaced by professionals and protocols". In their comprehensive report, they argue that the social determinants of dying and grieving should be tackled and that conversations about everyday death, dying and grieving should be commoner. AD is discussed and the majority of the 14 Lancet Commission authors who commented said that "AD should be part of end-of-life care", but their emphasis is on increasing death literacy and the family and community aspects of such care.[20]

In Section 7 of the Lancet Commission report, they discuss the literature on the will to live and the will to die, central issues in the consideration of the place of AD. They summarise the research that the "will to live" is affected by physical and psychological symptoms including pain, breathlessness and depression, but that it may be more affected by factors such as the loss of hope, feeling a burden or feeling that life has no meaning.[20, 22–23] Low scores on a will to love scoring system, correlated with breathlessness, absence of a spouse and high anxiety; high scores correlated with low anxiety and strong religious beliefs.[20, 22–24] Rodinet al.[25] noted that a cancer diagnosis could alter peoples will to live, but many cancer patients, even those with advanced disease, retain a strong will to survive their disease. In addressing the literature on the "will to hasten death", Rodriguez-Prat et al.,[26] conducted a meta-analysis of patients' experience. Access to good control of symptoms is a prominent positive influence on the will to live. Factors which reduced the will to live included pain, fatigue, breathlessness, problems with cognition, loss of independence, fear of the future and the process of dying, loss of self-determination and a wish to spare others from burdens.[26] Shimizu et al.[27] studied whether having a strong reason to live could influence the timing of death. They looked at a large number of death records in the USA and found that death rates were higher after Christmas and birthdays, suggesting that people may be able to postpone their deaths for a short time to have these important times with their loved ones.

In 2021, Zaman et al.[28] conducted a systematic review of literature on the factors which predicted for what they defined as "a good death" in 16 economically advantaged countries. Their findings were that the factors are relief of symptoms, effective communications with carers, performance of their religious and cultural rites, relief of distress, autonomy in decision making, choice of place of death, life not being prolonged unnecessarily, awareness of the significance of the event, support of family and friends, not being a burden and having the right to terminate their own life if they so choose.[28] In a setting of less wealth and less developed healthcare in Tanzania,[29] there were some similar findings but prioritising community and relatives above oneself, was highlighted.

The Lancet Commission highlighted that healthcare services at the end of life, are less often mentioned than others in policy and strategy documents, even though they often consume a large proportion of healthcare resources.[20] In their section on AD, the Lancet Commission summarise legal changes up to 2022 which will be updated in our later chapters. They emphasise the important of examining the international evidence on AD provide a useful checklist of the social, healthcare and policy issues as well as the legal ones.[20]

In our next chapters, we will review the legal debate and current Bills in the jurisdictions of the UK and the British Isles, the views of healthcare professionals and the international experience in jurisdictions which permit AD. Separate chapters will then review the impact of cultural and religious issues, the views and impact on disadvantaged and/or disabled people and the literature on patients and caregivers experience. Finally, we will summarise the place of AD in medical jurisprudence and attempt to draw some conclusions from the overall international experience.

Our focus will be on the current status and issues surrounding AD. However, we are all mindful that the social context reflected by the Lancet Commission and others, must also be considered in the wider debate about how societies approach death, dying and bereavement.

References

1. Board R, Bennett MI, Lewis P, et al., eds. End of life choices for cancer patients. An international perspective. Oxford: EBN Health, 2020.

2. Ring A, Harari D, Kalsi T, et al., eds. Problem solving in older cancer patients. Oxford: Clinical Publishing, 2016.

3. Copson E, Hall P, Board R, et al., eds. Problem solving through precision oncology. Oxford: Clinical Publishing, 2017.

4. Velikova G, Fallowfield L, Younger J, et al., eds. Problem solving in patient-centred and integrated cancer care. Oxford: EBN Health, 2018.

5. Board R, Nathan P, Newsom-Davis T, et al., eds. Problem solving in cancer immunotherapy. Oxford: EBN Health, 2019.

6. Young A, Board R, Leonard P, et al., eds. Problem solving in acute oncology (2nd edition). Oxford: EBN Health, 2020.

7. Karapanagiotou EM, Kopeika J, Board RE, et al., eds. Problem solving in cancer and fertility. Oxford: EBN Health, 2021.

8. Hickson S, Lee C, O'Cathail S, et al., eds. Problem solving in interventional oncology. Oxford: EBN Health, 2023.

9. Terminally Ill Adults (End of Life) Bill (As taken to the Lords). https://bills.parliament.uk/publications/61635/documents/6734; https://bills.parliament.uk/bills/3774/publications

10. Terminally Ill Adults (End of Life) Bill: impact assessment (updated). https://assets.publishing.service.gov.uk/media/68247bfdb9226dd8e81ab849/terminally-ill-adults-end-of-life-bill-impact-assessment-updated.pdf

11. Public and professional opinion on physician-assisted dying. https://www.bma.org.uk/media/ejcdado1/public-and-professional-opinion-on-pad-updated-jan-2025.pdf

12. British Social Attitudes 34 | Moral issues. Sex, gender identity and euthanasia. https://natcen. ac.uk/sites/default/files/2023-08/bsa34_moral_issues_final.pdf

13. Assisted dying principles, practice and politics. Complex Life and Death Decisions Group, The Policy Institute, Kings College London. October 2024. https://www.kcl.ac.uk/policy-institute/assets/14587oct-assisted-dying-survey-friday-4-oct.pdf

14. You Gov. Support for assisted dying unmoved by the debate. https://yougov.co.uk/health/ articles/52413-support-for-assisted-dying-unmoved-by-the-debate

15. YouGov survey results. https://ygo-assets-websites-editorial-mea.yougov.net/documents/ Internal_AssistedDying_250516_w.pdf

16. https://www.opinium.com

17. Opinium 2024. Will public opinion translate into legislative change? https://www.opinium. com/resource-center/will-public-opinion-translate-into-legislative-change

18. Ipsos Assisted Dying polling. Two thirds of UK public continue to think assisted dying should be legal, provided certain conditions are met. July 2023. https://www.ipsos.com/sites/ default/files/ct/news/documents/2023-08/ipsos-assisted-dying-survey-july-2023-charts.pdf

19. Bloomer MJ, Saffer L, Hewitt J, et al. Maybe for unbearable suffering: diverse racial, ethnic and cultural perspectives of assisted dying. A scoping review. Palliat Med. 2024;38(9):968–980.

20. Sallnow L, Smith R, Ahmedzai SH, et al. Lancet Commission on the Value of Death. Report of the Lancet Commission on the Value of Death: bringing death back into life. Lancet. 2022;399(10327):837–884.

21. Zaman M, Mohapatra A, Espinal-Arango S, et al. What would it take to die well? A systematic review of systematic reviews on the conditions for a good death. Lancet Healthy Longev. 2021;2:e593–e600.

22. Chochinov HM, Kristjanson LJ, Hack TF, et al. Burden to others and the terminally ill. J Pain Symptom Manage. 2007;34:463–71.

23. Tataryn D, Chochinov HM. Predicting the trajectory of will to live in terminally ill patients. Psychosomatics. 2002;43:370–377.

24. Khan L, Wong R, Li M, et al. Maintaining the will to live of patients with advanced cancer. Cancer J. 2010;16:524–531.

25. Rodin G, Zimmermann C, Rydall A , et al. The desire for hastened death in patients with metastatic cancer. J Pain Symptom Manage. 2007;33:661–675.

26. Rodríguez-Prat A, Balaguer A, Booth A, et al. Understanding patients' experiences of the wish to hasten death: an updated and expanded systematic review and meta-ethnography. BMJ Open. 2017;7:e016659.

27. Shimizu M, Pelham BW. Postponing a date with the Grim Reaper: ceremonial events and mortality. Basic Appl Soc Psych. 2008;30:36–45.

28. Zaman M, Mohapatra A, Espinal-Arango S, et al. What would it take to die well? A systematic review of systematic reviews on the conditions for a good death. Lancet Healthy Longev. 2021;2:e593–e600.

29. Gafaar TO, Pesambili M, Henke O, et al. Good death: an exploratory study on perceptions and attitudes of patients, relatives, and healthcare providers, in northern Tanzania. PLoS One. 2020;15:e0233494.

Chapter 2: The UK/British Isles Legal Debate

The legal debate on AD in England and Wales

At the time of writing, AD, whether in the form of assisted suicide or voluntary euthanasia, remains illegal in the UK in all jurisdictions.[1] However, in any year several dozen people from the UK travel abroad for assistance to die, principally to Switzerland. Doubts and uncertainties about the role of family members in helping them do so cause considerable anxiety. In February 2010, the Director of Public Prosecutions set out the factors to be considered when deciding whether a prosecution in an assisted suicide case is in the public interest. The policy suggests that it is unlikely to be in the public interest for a loved one who has assisted someone access to AD to be prosecuted, if the person who travelled to another jurisdiction for assistance with suicide had reached a voluntary, clear, settled and informed decision to do so, and the loved one who had helped them was wholly motivated by compassion.

In the UK Parliament, there have been attempts to change the law on AD for England and Wales since the 1930s, when a voluntary euthanasia bill was proposed. The Voluntary Euthanasia Society was formed in 1935. This society is now known as Dignity in Dying. Attempts at legal reform were made in 1936, 1969, 1976, 1990 and 1997 but were defeated. Lord Joffe introduced bills between 2003, 2004 and 2005 without success. Lord Falconer introduced an AD bill into the House of Lords in 2014, proposing that patients with a life expectancy of less than 6 months should have the choice of a medically assisted death, but it failed. In 2015, the MP Rob Marris brought forward a Private Member's Bill proposing assisted suicide, which was substantially based on Lord Falconer's proposals. The bill was defeated in the House of Commons in September 2015. In 2016, Lord Hayward introduced an AD bill in the Lords, but it did not progress (see 1).

The "Terminally Ill Adults (End of Life) Bill" was introduced to the UK Parliament (House of Commons, HoC) on October 2024 as Private Member's Bill (PMB) by Kim Leadbeater MP. The Bill passed its second reading in November 2024. This was debated passionately and approved by a majority of MPs. It has progressed through the Committee Stage and after amendments it has passed the third reading with a vote of 314 in favour and 291 against. It will progress to the House of Lords where it may well be further amended. The Bill in the amended form which has progressed to the House of Lords and the history of the Bill in Parliament are at Ref. 2 and the updated Impact Assessment is at Ref. 3. The Bill's first reading in the House of Lords was on the 23 June 2025. The Bill will have Committee and Report stages in the Lords before returning to the Commons for Consideration of Amendments after which, if passed, it will then receive Royal Assent for it to become a an Act of Parliament, that is, primary legislation.

The Bill refers to the proposed intervention as a "Voluntary Assisted Dying" (VAD) service. This is likely to become the term used for AD in the UK.

While it now seems likely that UK legislation to permit AD will be enacted in the foreseeable future, it is difficult to predict the timeline for implementation and access to assistance to die. For example, in Oregon the Death with Dignity Act was passed in 1994 but legal objections and delays meant it was not implemented until 1997. However long the process may be, it seems now appropriate for healthcare professionals in the disciplines closest to the patients who may choose AD, to have input into the refinement, planning and implementation of the Bill.

Provisions of the Terminally Ill Adults Bill

A convenient schematic, and clinically relevant, overview of the provisions of the Terminally Ill Adults Bill is given in Figure 2.1. At the time of writing, we are working from the Bill as it was taken to its first reading in the House of Lords[2] and the Impact statement of 14 May 2025.[3]

The Bill sets out a process for AD for terminally ill UK residents aged over 18 years who voluntarily, without any coercion or pressure, formed a clear, settled and informed wish to end their

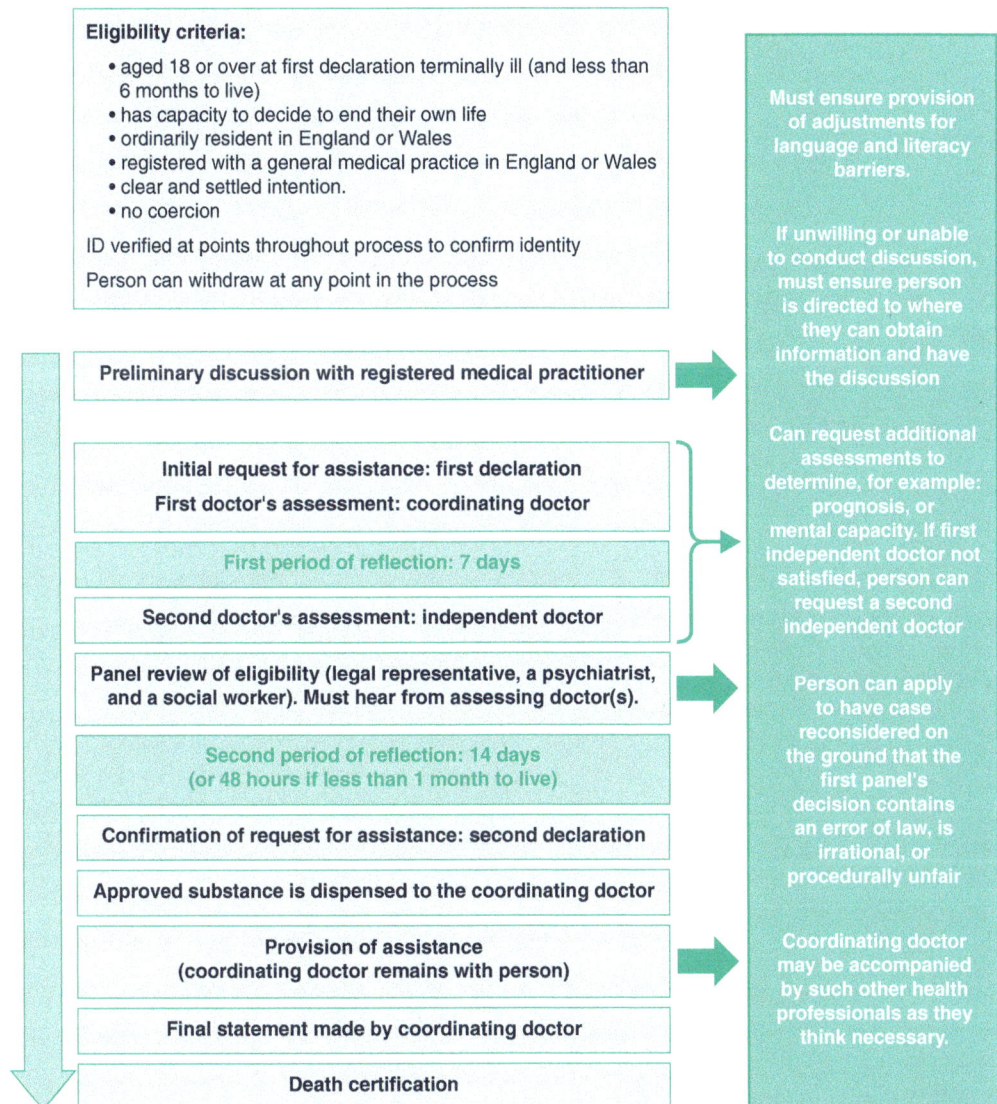

Eligibility criteria:
- aged 18 or over at first declaration terminally ill (and less than 6 months to live)
- has capacity to decide to end their own life
- ordinarily resident in England or Wales
- registered with a general medical practice in England or Wales
- clear and settled intention.
- no coercion

ID verified at points throughout process to confirm identity

Person can withdraw at any point in the process

Must ensure provision of adjustments for language and literacy barriers.

If unwilling or unable to conduct discussion, must ensure person is directed to where they can obtain information and have the discussion

Preliminary discussion with registered medical practitioner

Initial request for assistance: first declaration

First doctor's assessment: coordinating doctor

First period of reflection: 7 days

Second doctor's assessment: independent doctor

Can request additional assessments to determine, for example: prognosis, or mental capacity. If first independent doctor not satisfied, person can request a second independent doctor

Panel review of eligibility (legal representative, a psychiatrist, and a social worker). Must hear from assessing doctor(s).

Person can apply to have case reconsidered on the ground that the first panel's decision contains an error of law, is irrational, or procedurally unfair

Second period of reflection: 14 days (or 48 hours if less than 1 month to live)

Confirmation of request for assistance: second declaration

Approved substance is dispensed to the coordinating doctor

Provision of assistance (coordinating doctor remains with person)

Coordinating doctor may be accompanied by such other health professionals as they think necessary.

Final statement made by coordinating doctor

Death certification

Figure 2.1. Overview of the main steps an applicant would follow to access a VAD service in England or Wales.

own life. The person who has formed this wish must make a declaration to that effect witnessed by a coordinating doctor and another person aged over 18 years.

The eligibility requirements are therefore

- aged 18 or over at first declaration
- terminally ill (and a life expectancy estimated to be less than 6 months)
- has capacity to decide to end their own life
- ordinarily resident in England or Wales
- registered with a general medical practice in England or Wales
- clear, settled and informed intention to end their own life
- no evidence of coercion

ID will be verified throughout the process, and a person can withdraw at any point in the process.

The coordinating doctor is required to make assessments and be satisfied that the criteria for AD under the law are met and make a signed statement. This view must be supported by an independent doctor who must also be satisfied that the requirements are met.

The Bill as introduced included the requirement for the High Court to make a declaration that it is satisfied that the statutory criteria are met. This provision was amended during development of the Bill so this function will be provided by an expert panel. The panel would be appointed by a 'commissioner', who will be a sitting or retired senior judge.

The Bill defines a "terminal illness" as: (a) "…an inevitably progressive illness, disease or medical condition which cannot be reversed by treatment" and (b) "the person's death in consequence of that illness, disease or medical condition can reasonably be expected within 6 months."

Treatment which only relieves the symptoms of an inevitably progressive illness, disease or medical condition temporarily is not to be regarded as treatment which can reverse that illness or disease.

A person is not to be considered terminally ill only because they are a person with a disability or mental disorder (or both); however, having a disability or mental disorder does not prevent a person from being regarded as terminally ill if they meet the definition of terminally ill.

Two periods of reflection (7 days after the persons first declaration; 14 days after the panel's granting of a certificate of eligibility) are required. The person may cancel their declarations at any time. The coordinating doctor is required to make a second statement after the second period of reflection, that the person continues to meet the eligibility requirements of the bill.

AD is provided with an approved substance for self-administration. The coordinating doctor must stay with the person until they have self-administered the substance, and died, or the doctor determines that the procedure has failed.

The coordinating doctor makes a final statement that the person has died in accordance with the terms of the bill.

In summary (May 2025)[3] "**There is a three-stage approvals process**. The first is overseen by the "coordinating doctor", the second by an "independent doctor" and the third by a multidisciplinary "panel" comprised of a legal representative, psychiatrist, and social worker. At each stage, the doctor/panel must be satisfied that the person has a clear, settled and informed wish to end their own life, and has not been coerced or pressured by any other person into doing so.

Referral to an appropriate specialist can be made at each stage of the approvals process if there are doubts about the person's illness or mental capacity. This might include, for example, referral to a medical practitioner with expertise in the specific disease, condition, or illness in question, or to a psychiatrist or other health professional who has experience of assessing mental capacity.

The person must sign two written declarations to request an assisted death and can withdraw their consent at any time. Both declarations must be witnessed and recorded, alongside any notice of cancellations, in the person's medical records. A proxy can be appointed by the person if they are unable to sign their own name (by reason of physical impairment, being unable to read or for any other reason).

There are two 'periods of reflection' built into the process. The first period of reflection is 7 days between the first assessment by the coordinating doctor and second assessment by the independent doctor. The second period of reflection is 14 days (reducing to 48 hours if the person has less than 1 month to live) between the certificate of eligibility being granted by the panel and the provision of the approved substance.

The decision to self-administer the approved substance and final act of doing so must be taken by the person approved for an assisted death. The coordinating doctor (or another authorised practitioner) must remain with the person until their death is confirmed, before issuing the "final statement".

Each assisted death must be documented and reported for safety, monitoring and potential research purposes. Annual reports are to be published regarding implementation, and the legislation would undergo a review after 5 years.

Creation of new offences. Two new offences have been created to ensure safeguarding and correct processes. These pertain to 'dishonesty, coercion and pressure' and 'falsification or destruction of documents'.

Civil liability. A provision has been included to provide clarity that persons who are (i) providing assistance in accordance with the Bill, (ii) performing a function under the Bill or (iii) assisting a person in connection with doing of anything under the Bill, will not, of itself, give rise to a civil liability. It provides that civil liability can still arise where an act has been done dishonestly, or in some other way done otherwise than in good faith or breaches a duty of care owed to that person.

Free at point of access. The Bill requires the Secretary of State to, by regulations, make provision securing arrangements for the provision of VAD services in England and similarly provides Welsh Ministers with the power to make regulations about provision of VAD services in Wales. The Bill goes on to state that these regulations must state that such services are to be provided free of charge, except where charging is expressly provided for in relation to commissioned VAD services.

The Isle of Man

Isle of Man legislators have been at the forefront of the introduction of an Assisted Dying Bill with the Isle of Man Assisted Dying Bill 2023 (Private Members Bill) which was passed by Branches of the Tynwald in March 2025. This means that the Bill now awaits Royal Assent and is expected to become law in the foreseeable future making the island the first jurisdiction in the British Isles to legalise Assisted Dying. The Bill was debated in the Manx Parliament Legislative Council and the House of Keys. It went through a lengthy Committee stage, passing the final hurdles in 2025. The Isle of Man Medical Society was opposed to the Bill. The House of Keys voted in favour of final amendments. Its proposer was Alex Allinson, a GP and member of the House.[4–6]

The Bill allows terminally ill adults with a prognosis of 12 months or less to choose to end their lives, provided they meet specific criteria. This includes being over 18, registered with a

Manx GP, living on the island for 5 years, and having full mental capacity for this decision. The bill requires two independent doctors to assess the patient and confirm their eligibility. Following the assessment, a 14-day waiting period will be observed before an "approved substance" can be administered by a registered medical professional. The bill is expected to be in effect by 2027.[4-6]

Jersey

In May 2024, the Jersey States Assembly approved detailed proposals for AD in Jersey and requested the Minister for Health and Care, Jersey, to bring forward primary legislation that permits AD in Jersey for those with a terminal illness. It is anticipated that the earliest date the law would come into effect would be Summer 2027.[7]

The law is expected to set out the eligibility criteria for accessing assisted dying in Jersey. The eligibility criteria are expected to be:

- have been diagnosed with a terminal illness
- have decision-making capacity
- have a voluntary, settled and informed wish to end their own life
- be at least 18 years of age
- be ordinarily resident in Jersey for at least 12 months

No-one should be under a legal duty to participate directly in the provision of assisted dying, and they should have a right to refuse direct participation.

The Jersey Assisted Dying Service will be delivered by the Government of Jersey's Health and Care Jersey. A draft bill is expected by the end of 2025.[7-9]

Scotland

Liberal Democrat MSP Liam McArthur introduced the Assisted Dying for Terminally Ill Adults (Scotland) Bill in March 2024, which is under consideration by the Scottish Parliament.[10-12] Eligibility criteria include

- residence in Scotland for at least 12 months and registered with a GP in Scotland
- terminal illness
- mental capacity to make the request

For the Scottish Bill "For the purposes of this Act, a person is terminally ill if they have an advanced and progressive disease, illness or condition from which they are unable to recover and that can reasonably be expected to cause their premature death". Liam McArthur has proposed that the age for consent should be 18 years.

Members of the Scottish Parliament voted at stage one of their process in favour of the Bills general principles by 70 votes to 56, with one abstention, in May 2025.[11] There is now a process of amendments followed by a vote on the final draft. That process is expected to take several months. In October 2024, it was reported by the BBC that Scottish Health Secretary, Neil Gray, said the proposed legislation went beyond the limits of Holyrood's powers and was a matter for Westminster. However, Mr McArthur said he was confident the UK and Scottish governments could find a solution if MSPs backed his bill.[10-12]

Table 2.1

Jurisdiction	Status	Eligibility criteria (Life expectancy)
UK/E&W	Pending	<6 m
Isle of Man	Pending	<12 m
Jersey	Pending	<6m (<12 m Neuro Degen Dis)
Scotland	Pending	Terminal Diagnosis

Patients from all UK jurisdictions travelling to Switzerland

The potential impact of changes in the UK legislation on AD UK-residents who travel to Switzerland to access AD was studied by Brewer et al.[13] They collected information from the main organisations offering AD in Switzerland on UK patients. For comparison, they used data from Oregon which has since 1997 had similar legislation to that proposed for the UK. The differences between UK residents travelling to Switzerland and the Oregon patient population are substantial. For example, while 72.5% of Oregon patients had cancer, only 22.7% of UK residents who travelled to Switzerland had such a diagnosis. 49.6% of UK patients travelling to Switzerland had a neurological condition compared to only 11.2% of patients accessing AD in Oregon. Many of the patients with neurological conditions were felt to have a prognosis of more than 6 months and would not have been eligible for AD under proposed UK legislation .[13]

Conclusions

It will be immediately apparent that the UK debate on Assisted Dying has been prolonged, complex and challenging. Different UK and British Isles jurisdictions have and are still progressing laws which are somewhat different from each other (Table 2.1). Public opinion as measured in surveys over a long period of time seems to be stably and consistently supportive of a change in the law to allow some form of Assisted Dying. In the last few years, the opinion of legislators in all the jurisdictions that are active in the process of legislation now, seems to have shifted towards support for a change in the law, but the level of support is often less than the recorded public support for change.

In the next chapters in this book, we will describe and evaluate the experience of legislating for and delivering Assisted Dying worldwide, to inform and support the UK public, their legislators and professionals about what has been learned that may help the process in the UK. We are mindful of the advice issued in the UK by the Chief Medical Officers of the nations of the UK:

"This has to be a decision for society as a whole, expressed through Parliament.

Whatever Parliament decides, we believe the medical profession will be unanimous on 2 things:

- *that we must not undermine the provision of good end-of-life care for all including the outstanding work done by palliative care clinicians*
- *that individual doctors and other healthcare workers should be able to exercise freedom of conscience as, for example, happens with abortion care currently*

This will, we are sure, be common ground for all sides of this complex societal decision".[14]

References

1. Board R, Bennett MI, Lewis P, et al., eds. End of life choices for cancer patients. An international perspective. Oxford: EBN Health, 2020.

2. Terminally Ill Adults (End of Life) Bill (as taken to the Lords). https://bills.parliament.uk/publications/61635/documents/6734; https://bills.parliament.uk/bills/3774/publications

3. Terminally Ill Adults (End of Life) Bill: impact assessment (updated). https://assets.publishing.service.gov.uk/media/68247bfdb9226dd8e81ab849/terminally-ill-adults-end-of-life-bill-impact-assessment-updated.pdf

4. Isle of Man Assisted Dying Bill 2023 (Private Members Bill) Passed by the Branches. https://tynwald.org.im/business/bills

5. House of Keys Committee on the Assisted Dying Bill Report. https://tynwald.org.im/spfile?file=/business/bills/Bills/2024-PP-0048.pdf

6. Iacobucci G. Isle of Man poised to legalise assisted dying after vote. BMJ. 2025;388.

7. Assisted dying in Jersey. https://www.gov.je/Caring/AssistedDying/pages/assisteddying.aspx

8. Iacobucci G. Jersey is set to allow assisted dying. BMJ 2021;375.

9. Assisted dying plans for terminally ill approved. https://www.bbc.co.uk/news/articles/c6ppl7e551do

10. Assisted Dying for Terminally Ill Adults (Scotland) Bill [AS INTRODUCED]. https://www.parliament.scot/-/media/files/legislation/bills/s6-bills/assisted-dying-for-terminally-ill-adults-scotland-bill/introduction/bill-as-introduced.pdf

11. Christie B. Assisted dying bill clears first hurdle in Scotland BMJ. 2025;389.

12. How could assisted dying laws change? https://www.bbc.co.uk/news/uk-47158287

13. Brewer C, Hopwood MC, Winyard G. Assisted deaths in Switzerland for UK residents: diagnoses and their implications for palliative medicine and assisted dying legislation. BMJ Support Palliat Care. 2024;0:1–3. spcare-2023-004719.

14. UK chief medical officers and NHS England National Medical Director. Assisted Dying debate: advice to doctors. 2024. https://www.gov.uk/government/publications/assisted-dying-bill-debate-advice-to-doctors

Chapter 3: Views of UK Healthcare Professionals

The majority of people requesting some form of AD worldwide have a cancer diagnosis and all healthcare professionals (HCPs) need to be able to have open conversations with patients about choices at the end of life. It is vital to understand how HCPs feel about this debate, what their role may be in any change to legislation and potential challenges and practicalities that should be considered.

Oncologists, in particular, are well versed in holding frank and open conversations with patients and their carers about treatment options and prognosis. Often these conversations are difficult, dealing with uncertainty and raw emotions. Towards the end of life these conversations, as shared decision making continues, the focus shifts subtly to establishing goals on end-of-life care, hopes for the future, preferred place of care at the end of life and determining what a "good death" might look like for that individual. For the majority of patients these conversations will ultimately lead to peaceful and dignified dying.

Occasionally patients may request AD. Often these are cries for help, born out of frustration, anger or due to the suffering of an as yet uncontrolled symptom. But sometimes patients have a clear wish for control over the date and timing of their own death. Current legislation in the UK rules physician AD or euthanasia to be illegal. However, with the current proposed changes to legislation this position may change in the near future.

The Association of Cancer Physicians/UK Society for Medical Oncology is recognised by the Royal College of Physicians (RCP) and the Department of Health as the specialty association for medical oncologists. They perform several functions including promoting the views and interests of medical oncologists, influencing policy on cancer care and consultant expansion, assisting in the development of training curricula and the specialty examination and participation in NICE appraisals and national guideline development.

In 2019, the ACP held a workshop on Assisted Dying, where there was a consensus that the decision to change the law to permit AD in the UK must be made by society and its legislators rather than by medical disciplines. The ACP position is therefore neutral, as is that of the RCP. The ACP position is given in Box 3.1.

Opinion of UK oncologists

The Royal College of Physicians (RCP) is a professional body in the UK representing physicians across the globe. Practising medical oncologists in the UK are required to pass the RCP membership (MRCP) exams in order to secure approval for training in medical oncology, the most common training pathway to become a UK consultant in medical oncology. In early 2019, the RCP polled its membership of over 35,000 doctors to gather their views on AD. The online survey, carried out between 5 February and 1 March 2019 was completed by 6885 respondents from more than 30 medical specialties.

The following questions were asked of members:

What should the RCP's position be on whether or not there should be a change in the law to permit AD? In favour 31.6%. Opposed 43.4%. Neutral 25.0%

Box 3.1   Position statement on assisted dying.

The Association of Cancer Physicians/UK Society for Medical Oncology

The Association of Cancer Physicians/UK Society for Medical Oncology is recognised by the Royal College of Physicians (RCP) and the Department of Health as the specialty association for medical oncologists. We:

- Care for cancer patients and deliver medical cancer treatment often as part of multidisciplinary teams.
- Encourage the development of best practice to benefit patients.
- Promote the views and interests of medical oncologists.
- Influence policy on cancer care and consultant expansion.
- Assist in the development of training curricula and the specialty examination.
- Participate in NICE appraisals and guideline development.

In this Position Statement we use the term "assisted dying" (AD) to refer to the assistance of a person to deliberately end their own life. In the UK, AD is the term referred to in most applications for legal change. We acknowledge that AD is also used to refer to both assisted suicide (a person self-administers lethal medications to end their own life) and euthanasia (a person administers lethal medications to end another person's life).

In 2019 the ACP held a workshop on Assisted Dying, where there was a consensus that the decision to change the law to permit AD in the UK must be made by society and its legislators rather than by medical disciplines. The ACP position is therefore neutral, as is that of the RCP. Surveys of Medical Oncologists show a range of individual opinions on legal change, without a majority for or against.

The ACP notes

- Recent surveys suggest the majority of UK citizens consulted support a change in the law to permit very carefully regulated AD.
- The first vote in the UK Parliament on a bill to permit AD was supportive of change.
- Protection of vulnerable patients is a priority for the ACP and all healthcare professionals.
- Most medical oncologists, as other doctors, have indicated that they would not take an active role in the delivery of AD.
- There should not be any assumption that AD will be a doctor's responsibility.
- Estimates of prognosis are frequently inaccurate and must be used with extreme caution.
- There is a need for additional training for the medical oncology workforce around AD, including the ethical and legal issues.

Do you support a change in the law to permit AD? Yes 40.5%. No 49.1%. Undecided 10.4%

Regardless of your support or opposition to change, if the law was changed to permit AD, would you be prepared to participate actively? Yes 24.6%. No 55.1%. Don't know 20.3%

In response to this poll the RCP dropped its opposition to changing the law on AD and took a neutral stance. The RCP president at the time of the survey Professor Andrew Goddard said: "*It is clear that there is a range of views on AD in medicine, just as there is in society. We have been open from the start of this process that adopting a neutral position will mean that we can reflect the differing opinions among our membership. Neutral means the RCP neither supports nor opposes a change in the law and we won't be focusing on AD in our work. Instead, we will continue championing high-quality palliative care services."*

In should be noted that whilst there was no consensus view for the majority of specialities, palliative care physicians voted clearly that the RCP should be opposed to a change in the law on AD.[1-3]

The Royal College of Radiologists (RCR) represents radiologists and clinical oncologists in the UK. In the UK, clinical oncologists deliver a substantial proportion of systemic medicine-based treatment for cancer and all radiotherapy. In February 2019, the RCR polled the 1572 UK clinical oncology members and fellows to gain insight into the views of clinical oncologist members on AD. The questions mirrored the RCP survey. Results of 532 valid survey responses were presented, and the conclusion was that "the results of this survey show that opinion varies across the faculty of clinical oncology, as would be expected. We do not intend to hold an official Faculty of Clinical Oncology position on AD but will make these results available publicly".[4]

Comparisons of responses between medical and clinical oncologists show very little variation between the two groups and no significant differences in opinion when compared to the RCP results as a whole.

What should the Colleges' position be on whether or not there should be a change in the law to permit AD?

Medical Oncology.	In favour 31.85%	Opposed 37.15%	Neutral 31.05%
Clinical Oncology.	In favour 26.90%	Opposed 30.30%	Neutral 42.90%

Do you support a change in the law to permit AD?

Medical Oncology.	Yes 42.07%	No 47.95%	Undecided 9.35%
Clinical Oncology.	Yes 37.30%	No 46.90%	Undecided 16.00%

If the law was changed to permit AD, would you be prepared to participate actively?

Medical Oncology.	Yes 24.65%	No 58.80%	Undecided 16.50%
Clinical Oncology.	Yes 23.20%	No 56.10%	Undecided 20.90%

Considerations for oncologists

Workforce

The current proposed bill in England requires a coordinating doctor and an independent doctor to assess the patient. There is currently a national shortage of oncology physicians with a 15% shortage of clinical oncologists projected to rise to 21% by 2028. This, together with increasing complexity and number of systemic anti-cancer therapies and radiotherapy treatments, means the pressure on the oncology workforce is rising all the time, leading to delays in patients' treatments. As >50% of patients accessing AD in other countries have a cancer diagnosis, oncologists are likely to be required to play a role in assessment and coordination of this service. Significant attention needs to be given to how oncologists could be expected to participate in these services whilst still providing an optimal non-surgical oncology provision, especially as the RCP and RCR surveys reported that less than a quarter of oncologists would be happy to actively participate. The tight timelines around the provision of AD could lead to conflict between providing a timely service for patients on treatment and assessing and providing these services. Specialist high quality oncology and end of life care for all is an NHS commitment.

If the law were changed to AD, a dedicated AD service would need to be developed. Any such service would need additional funding and should be multiprofessional and not be at the expense of funding for cancer screening, diagnostics, treatments and importantly palliative and supportive care.

Prognosis

The Bill defines a 'terminal illness' as: '(a)…an inevitably progressive illness, disease or medical condition which cannot be reversed by treatment' and (b) the person's death in consequence of that illness, disease or medical condition can reasonably be expected within 6 months'.

Determining prognosis in oncology is notoriously contentious and changes over time. For example, <5% of patients with metastatic melanoma in 2015 would be expected to survive 5 years but that figure is now over 50% in 2024 for those patients with access to best standard of care immunotherapy. Whilst there are some clinical parameters that can aid prognostication such as performance status, and some pathology results such as low protein and low Hb, clinicians in fact tend to overestimate prognosis. In general, the accuracy of prediction for patient survival is better when the estimate is made near death, whereas prognostication over a longer term seems more uncertain. In the context of AD, this provides significant challenges for clinicians – does one risk overestimation and find the patient deteriorates more quickly with insufficient time to receive AD as per their wishes, or wait till there is more certainty and again risk the patient being too unwell to fulfil their wishes? Conversely, if a patient given less than 6 months to live proceeds with AD, what is the impact on the clinician and family if novel treatments with high success become available after the patient's death?

It is possible statistical tools and AI based algorithms may allow for better prediction of survival in the future, but until then, that responsibility appears to fall firmly and squarely on the shoulders of clinicians. For oncologists, the increasing specialisation of cancers and their treatments could lead to a small number of specialists taking the task to assess patients requesting AD, especially in the case of rarer tumours, in order to try and better prognosticate for these patient groups. Treleaven et al.[5] carried out a systematic review of the literature on the limitations on the accuracy of prognosis. The prognostic tools added relatively little to the accuracy of prognosis. They were better predicting shorter prognosis

The approach taken in some jurisdictions to indicate that the estimation of prognosis should be articulated on the balance of probabilities, seems sensible. So, the appropriate clinicians would be asked to say that "on the balance of probabilities a person may die within 6 months", for example.

Psychological impact on the clinicians

Physicians are trained to preserve and prolong the life of patients by curing illnesses and to "do no harm". Physicians who receive a request for AD may experience a conflict of duties and morals: the duty to preserve life on the one hand and the duty to relieve suffering on the other. The psychological burden of both the decision making for eligibility, especially with uncertainties around prognosis, and, the involvement in the prescribing of the "approved substance for self-administration" with a need to accompany the patient at the time of administration, should not be underestimated.

For oncologists openly involved in any AD assessments or services there is little known about how this may impact on their relationship with colleagues and other staff, and some may be concerned about the reaction of those in the wider population who have strong views opposed to AD. There could be an associated impact on occupational health and mental wellbeing services which need to be able to support any clinicians, other healthcare professionals, managerial and administrative staff involved in the patients' pathway. Looking to countries where AD is legal it is clear that there is a significant and complex emotional burden on clinicians preparing and performing AD. Some clinicians may feel pressure to approve requests when they felt eligibility wasn't fulfilled. Contradictory and conflicting emotions were experienced by the majority of Dutch clinicians involved reported by Evenblij et al.,[6] Wibisono et al.,[7] Winters et al.[8] and Winters et al.[9] found mixed impacts on Canadian physicians with some reporting great satisfaction in contributing to the relief of suffering in the AD/MAiD process but some feeling conflicted. There was no evidence of an excess of mental health issues among physicians participating in AD in a systematic review.[7] The psychological wellbeing and mental health of all involved in AD needs to be supported and monitoring and further research in this area is indicated.

Impact on the patient–doctor relationship

Involvement in AD could have an impact on the relationship of a doctor with their patient and those important to the patient such as families and care givers. The nature and extent of the impact would depend on the level and nature of involvement of the doctor. Where conscientious objection is exercised, the patient may not be offered access to AD, and if they do assess the service, they may have to form another relationship with a clinician who will ultimately be present at the time of their death and not the oncologist they have known for potentially many years. Equally, patients could feel a pressure to discuss AD or a concern that this would be forced on them by oncologists openly involved in these services. This could lead to them not being as honest with their doctor about symptoms and concerns out of fear of being offered AD. Oncologists and palliative care clinicians involved in care for patients at the end of life will need to carefully negotiate the way through this new world.

The RCP released a further position statement on 2025,[3] confirming their neutral position and outline key factors they feel should be included in legislation including the need for equitable choice, difficulties around assessment of prognosis, lack of multidisciplinary assessment, need for more regulation for capacity and safeguarding, Patients must be enabled to have an equitable choice of services as they approach the end of their lives and the need for more clarity around what will be included in secondary legislation for example. Training, regulation, and qualifications. They state, "*Assisted dying services must not divert resources from other end of life care which must be available for all patients, or disadvantage provision of end of life and other services*".[3]

Assisted dying – what do UK Palliative Care Doctors think and what could be the impact of assisted dying be on them?

Oncologists and Palliative Medicine specialists work very closely together, and oncologists seek to ensure as much early engagement of patients with Palliative Care as possible within available capacity. Much of this joint work relates to care for patients at the end of life. However, it is important to point out that the expertise of Palliative Care specialists in symptom management, such as pain relief, is also very relevant to patients who are on treatment programmes aimed at cure. They may also benefit in terms of their quality of life and outcomes from Palliative care input and expertise. The views of oncologists and palliative care healthcare professionals are closely related to each other and there have been close interrelationships between oncological and palliative care services over many years.

The professional organisations which represent the two professional groups do have different positions on AD set out in their Position Statements in Boxes 3.1 and 3.2. However, the dialogue between them is an ongoing and open one which will become of considerable importance should a change in UK law to permit assisted dying be made. There is a consensus supported actively by all oncologists that the provision of high quality and well-resourced palliative care is central to the care of cancer patients throughout their journey.

A clear majority of the members of the Association for Palliative Medicine of Great Britain and Ireland (APM) are against the legalisation of Assisted Dying (10, Box 3.2). This is the basis for the stance of the APM opposing a change in the law. Individual palliative medicine physicians also contribute regularly and consistently to national debate in the media and reflect the diversity of opinion across the specialty. Stated opposition to assisted dying is often grounded in concerns regarding the context of implementation.

Other oncology and surgery contributors to this paper have already considered potential impacts on doctor-patient relationships, including aspects of capacity and coercion, priorities within clinical services, and the impact on practitioner emotional well-being. Such impacts resonate with palliative care and, along with challenges in accurate prognostication, will not be covered again in detail here. Likewise, the nature of healthcare as a multiprofessional and multidisciplinary team endeavour has been well described, and contrasts with a TIA Bill that places so much focus on assessment and delivery by individual doctors, The implications of assisted suicide being considered as a medical treatment – as a therapy – are also highly pertinent to palliative care. In its position statement, the APM states three main grounds for opposing assisted dying:

Protection of vulnerable, frail, elderly, disabled and terminally ill people

It is of note that the professional associations representing doctors in closest proximity to frail, elderly, and terminally ill people – GPs, geriatricians and palliative care physicians – report higher proportions of members opposed to assisted dying. The limitations to effective safeguarding, particularly in relation to vulnerability to coercion, and limitations to capacity, of many people towards the end of life are key concerns.

Direct coercion is recognised, and safeguarding processes are in place in health and social care, to protect those vulnerable to coercion. For example, the one in six over 65's who have experienced elder abuse.[11] More challenging is the detection and evidencing of indirect coercion, which may be due to perceptions of self and societal expectations; other social factors, and within the doctor-patient relationship.

Feeling a burden on others is a frequent reason for requesting AD and raises concern about more indirect social coercion. We are familiar with the particular challenges of those at the end of life who are vulnerably housed or homeless, and on incomes insufficient to meet the hidden costs of being cared for at home, or visited by their relatives in hospital, or for whom access to health and social care is limited either due to barriers to access to, or lack of availability of, services.

The AD debate has highlighted the low level of death literacy in our communities, which impacts on the choices people make. Death literacy influences the support available to people and their carers towards the end of life, as well as how trustworthy they perceive health care professionals and services to be. Reassurance is needed that in clinical experience, effective pain relief and other symptom management neither hasten nor postpone death. Likewise, where the burdens of continued medical treatment outweigh the benefits, a decision to stop this treatment may be made, either at the request of a patient with capacity, or on a best interests' basis for people who lack capacity for treatment decisions. Awareness of normal dying, characterised by the body shutting down, is limited. People may consider AD out of fear of a painful and distressing death, unaware that with attentive palliative care, be this pre-emptive surgery to prevent symptoms from mechanical causes; oncological therapy to reduce pressure or systemic effects, or expert medical symptom management, distressing deaths are the exception.

Fluctuating mental and physical capacity is very common in late-stage illness, due to the compounding factors of underlying physiological processes, fatigue, medication and feeling overwhelmed. There are two main concerns associated with this in relation to AD. Firstly, there is a concern that people may decide in favour of AD whilst incapacitated and doctors do at times make incorrect assessments of individuals' decision-making capacity. Secondly, symptom-relieving medication may be declined by individuals seeking AD in the fear that it may impair their capacity to complete the necessary legal processes, leaving them open to sub-optimal symptom management, as discussed by Hitchens.[12,13]

Box 3.2 **Position statement on assisted dying.**

The Association for Palliative Medicine

The Association for Palliative Medicine of Great Britain and Ireland (APM) is one of the world's largest representative bodies of medical/healthcare professionals practicing or interested in Palliative Medicine with a membership of over 1400.

In this Position Statement we use the term "assisted dying" (AD) to refer to the assistance of a person to deliberately end their own life. In the UK, AD is the term referred to in most applications for legal change. We acknowledge that AD is also used to refer to both assisted suicide (a person self-administers lethal medications to end their own life) and euthanasia (a person administers lethal medications to end another person's life).

The APM opposes any change in the law that could lead to the supply or administration of lethal medications to deliberately end a person's life.

The APM's position is supported by the consistent findings of multiple surveys:

2015. APM members survey – 82% were opposed to changing the law on Assisted Suicide.

2019. Royal College of Physicians – stratified for palliative medicine – 84.3% oppose a change in the law, and 84.4% were not prepared to actively participate in physician assisted suicide.

2020. British Medical Associations – stratified for palliative medicine – 70% were opposed to a change in the law and 84% would not be willing to actively participate in the process of prescribing life-ending drugs.

2022. APM Scotland survey – 75% of Scottish APM members responding would not be willing to participate in any part of the AD process and 98% stated that AD should not be part of mainstream healthcare.

The APM acknowledges that, while a substantial majority of APM members oppose AD, some of our members have a different view. The APM opposes the legislation of AD because of concerns about:

1. Protection of vulnerable, frail, elderly, disabled and terminally ill people.

2. The lack of adequately funded and equally available specialist palliative care services in all areas in the UK.

3. Concerns about trust and the impact on doctor-patient relationships.

The lack of adequately funded and equally available specialist palliative care services in all areas of the UK

Due to historical factors, there is wide variability in the availability and configuration of palliative care services. Specialist palliative care provision across all settings may be wholly or partially funded to varying degrees by the NHS and/or charity with both sources facing significant financial pressures, ever-increasing demand, and workforce constraints. Access is also inequitable, particularly to inpatient hospice care. The urgent need to address the resourcing of palliative care services was recognised by the House of Commons Health and Social Care Committee (HSC) in their Enquiry on Assisted Dying/Assisted Suicide and By the Marie Curie Better End of Life 2024 Report,[14,15] and, subsequently The Health Secretary, Wes Streeting, declared that it was his personal view that now was not the time to pursue a change in legislation as palliative care was 'not fit for purpose'.[16]

Therefore, currently, the reality of choice in end-of-life care for many is restricted due to barriers to access of existing services or gaps in provision. In a closed system with finite resources which are already pressurised, the ethical question then arises of how resources can be used to have the greatest impact on choice and experience for all people at the end of life. An NHS funded assisted dying/suicide service will not be cheap to deliver, and although there may be savings in other parts of the NHS, transferring savings in a cash strapped service is difficult and there is concern that an AD service will come at the expense of services elsewhere. This is a significant concern for those working in palliative care which is already facing severe financial pressures. The House of Commons HSC found that introducing AD did not negatively impact on Palliative Care Services.[14] However, Jones[17] argues that recent evidence suggests that increased investment in Palliative Care has been less in jurisdictions with AD than in those without AD.[17]

Another source of concern is the potential for funding for palliative care services to be linked to opting in to the provision of assisted dying. Kim Leadbeater is keen for all end-of-life care services including assisted dying to be provided 'holistically', and amendments to enable hospices and care homes to opt-out or set a policy of not providing AD, were denied by the Leadbeater Committee. There is also no guarantee that service providers will not lose public funding for not offering assisted suicide. This would have significant impact on the hospice sector, particularly those with religious statutes preventing involvement with AD. This is particularly relevant for oncology, as people with cancer are more likely to access inpatient hospice care and to die in hospices compared to people with noncancer diagnoses.

Concerns about trust and the impact on the doctor–patient relationship

As described earlier by oncology colleagues, subtle and unintended coercion may arise within a therapeutic relationship. For example, a doctor highlighting the availability of AD to a patient could influence their perception of AD as being a relevant option for them or suggest that the doctor believes that their dying will be distressing. Conversely, a patient may view the recommendations of a doctor known to favour legalised AD with caution, and perhaps be wary, for example, that a prescription for symptom relief might shorten their life. Mistrust of palliative care is already known to restrict access for minority ethnic groups, and this may be compounded by the availability of AD, particularly if it is provided within routine clinical care. The balance here is difficult. There is the risk of undue influence if legislation permits doctors to raise the option of AD, however there is a tension and discontinuity with usual practice if doctors are prohibited from raising all potential options.[18]

The APM believes that the ability to make a conscientious objection to participating in assisted dying is essential for both individuals and organisations. However, the TIA Bill does not outline true conscientious objection, which would include being able to refuse onward referral for AD. As mentioned previously, the amendment (481) denying hospices and care homes the right to opt out, and the lack of guarantee that they won't lose public funding, are significant and will impact the shape of hospice provision. Some Palliative care doctors are also concerned that, as many hospice organisations are neutral in the legalisation of AD debate, there may an expectation of their involvement should the Bill be passed. Many have said that they would resign if placed in this position.

The ongoing debate on the legalisation of AD has raised awareness of the complexity of questions related to death and dying and the current gaps in palliative care provision. There is an urgent need to ensure equity of access to high quality palliative care both now, and into an immediate future where the demographic 'bulge' is already rapidly escalating demand on health and social care. AD should only be considered within a society and healthcare system where high-quality palliative care is universally accessible in all settings of care, is fully funded and sufficiently resourced.

Views and opinions other UK Royal Colleges

In January 2025, the British Medical Association reviewed publications on professional opinion on Physician Assisted Dying.[19] Reports from the Royal College of Physicians (2019) and the Royal College of Radiologists' Faculty of Clinical Oncology (2019) are considered above. Updated views from other UK colleges are outlined below.

In October 2024, the **Royal College of Psychiatrists** (RCPsych) surveyed their members in England, Wales and Northern Ireland about the current proposed Bill. Members were asked their views on proposed legislation which would allow doctors to prescribe drugs for self-administration by a person aged >18, with a terminal illness, who had capacity and had given valid consent. The responses were "Opposed or strongly opposed" 44.8%; "Supported or strongly supported" 44.7%. In Scotland, the question was slightly different, "What is your general view about AD/assisted suicide for eligible terminally ill adults as defined in the Bill (those with "an advanced and progressive disease, illness or condition from which they are unable to recover and that can reasonably be expected to cause their premature death.") and the responses were Strongly or broadly in favour 45%; Strongly or broadly opposed 41%. The RCPsych does not have a formal position on AD but warns that terminal illness is a risk factor for suicide and remains concerned that a treatable mental illness could be a cause for a person wanting to end their life.

The proposed AD legislation in its current form as per July 2025, states that the assessing doctor must, "if they have doubt as to the capacity of the person being assessed, refer the person for assessment by a registered medical practitioner who is a practising psychiatrist registered in 1 of the 35 psychiatry specialisms in the Specialist Register kept by the General Medical Council or who otherwise holds qualifications in or has experience of the assessment of capacity". Furthermore, the Assisted Dying Review Panel, who's function it is to confirm eligibility to be provided with assistance must contain a psychiatrist member. Hence Psychiatrists will form an essential part of any AD service. Data from RCPsych shows that 58% of respondents said they would not be willing to participate, including determinations of capacity or assessing for mental disorder. With only 30% of respondents willing to participate if AD becomes legal in the UK, similarly to other medical specialities, lack of workforce able or willing to contribute to an AD service could be a barrier to implementation.

Other issues of concern for RCPsych are also worth mentioning especially as the college remain unconvinced that the most recent bill provides sufficient safeguards for patients with mental illness or those vulnerable to coercion. Some of the specific concerns include: the lack of provision for a holistic assessment of unmet need including intolerable pain, and social factors such as housing and finances; legal implications around the ambiguity of whether AD is considered a treatment option; the lack of a framework for assessing decisions about ending one's own life in the current Mental Capacity Act; clarity around the role of psychiatrists in the process and on the panel; and they ask for acknowledgment that physical effects of a mental disorder e.g. dementia or anorexia, shouldn't make a person eligible for assisted dying/assisted suicide.[20]

In March 2025, the UK Council of **Royal College of General Practitioners** (RCGP) moved to a position of neither supporting nor opposing assisted dying being legal, having been previously opposed following a 2019 vote. A survey of 8779 members revealed 33.7% believed the RCGP should support assisted dying being legal (subject to appropriate regulatory framework and safeguarding processes), 47.6% believed the RCGP should be opposed, 13.6% believed the RCGP should be neutral with 5.1% undecided.

Responding to the council's decision Professor Kamila Hawthorne, Chair of the Royal College of GPs, said: *"Today's discussion and our recent survey of our members, have clearly shown that GPs have widely differing and strongly held views about assisted dying – we care deeply about our patients. This is a highly sensitive personal, societal and legislative issue, and we need to be in a position to represent the views of all of our members and patients; shifting to a position of neither opposing nor supporting assisted dying being legal will allow us to do this best.*

"Neither opposing nor supporting assisted dying does not mean we will be stepping back from the debate. Our focus will be on advocating for our members, regardless of their views on assisted dying, as to how potential changes in the law will impact on their daily practice and the care they deliver for patients."

The college state that they will continue to engage with the legislative debate to ensure that any changes to the law protect the interests of all patients and healthcare professionals, and that palliative care is appropriately resourced.

Should there be a change in the law to permit assisted dying the RCCP website states:

- it should be seen as an additional specialised service that GPs and other healthcare professionals may opt to provide with additional training, and not part of core general practice.
- it should be a standalone service that will need to be separately and adequately resourced.
- there should be a right to refuse to participate in the process on any ground and statutory protection making it unlawful to discriminate against, or cause detriment to, any doctor on the basis of their decision to, or not to participate in the assisted dying process.
- work should be undertaken to define standards and training for those involved in delivering assisted dying services; and crucially
- it should not have a negative impact on funding for palliative care services in any way.

Professor Hawthorne concludes *"When patients are at or near the ends of their lives it is often when they need the most care, support and time from their healthcare professionals. Above all else, it is vital that regardless of whether or not assisted dying is permitted for terminally ill patients, they have access to the best possible palliative and end of life care".*[21]

In addition to medical oncologists and clinical oncologists, **surgeons** can play important roles in the care of terminally ill patients. Whilst surgical oncologists are most directly involved in the care of cancer patients, even surgeons who do not specialise in cancer are often involved, because terminally ill patients may have emergency admissions to hospital, for example, bowel obstruction in patients with metastatic and incurable colonic cancer. In 2014, the **Council of the Royal College of Surgeons (RCS)** of England had decided to oppose AD.[22] In 2021, the College decided to reconsider its position, and it commissioned Enventure Research, an independent research agency, to conduct a survey of its UK-based membership. An online survey of 17,361 members was conducted during February and March 2023, with a 19% response. Two main questions in the survey elicited the following responses:

- What RCS England's position should be towards a change in the law to permit doctors to supply drugs to qualifying patients to self-administer to end their own life?
  Responses: 52% supportive; 20% neutral; 25% opposed; 3% undecided
- What their (the member surgeons) personal position is towards a change in the law to permit doctors to supply drugs to qualifying patients to self-administer to end their own life, and the reasons for this position?

Responses: 61% supportive; 29% opposed; 10% undecided

When asked to explain their views, the most common reasons given were that patients should have choice/autonomy/control (39%) and that patients should not have to suffer/experience poor quality of life (38%). However, there were substantial comments to identify the need for clear safeguards (20%), protect vulnerable patients (15%), that doctors should do no hard (12%), the importance of personal/religious beliefs among doctors (11%) and that there should be a focus on Palliative care (11%). Following the survey,[23] the Council has voted to change the College's position to neutral from its earlier opposition to AD.

In July 2024, the **Royal College of Anaesthetists** asked its members the question "What should the position of the Royal College of Anaesthetists be on a change in the law allowing doctors to prescribe drugs for eligible patients to self-administer to end their own life?". The responses were "Supportive" 49%; "Opposed" 17% and "Neutral" 29%. This led to a change in the College's position from 'no stance' to 'neutral', meaning that the College neither actively supports nor actively opposes a change in the law. However, the College is now able to engage in discussion on the topic, which the previous 'no stance' position did not allow.[24]

The **Royal College of Pathologists (RCPath)** has no position on the ethical issues relating to assisted dying and recognises that its members hold a range of views. However, the RCPath has concerns about clause 35 in the bill as currently proposed that would prevent death following AD from requiring notification to the coroner. All AD deaths would be scrutinised by a medical examiner, but the opinion of the RCPath is that deaths following assisted dying should be notified to the coroner, just as other deaths following the administration of drugs, prescribed or not, must be. This concerns stems from the fact that medical examiners (who are members of RCPath) would need to review the process leading up to the decision of AD and the circumstances around the AD, and they are not qualified to do so. The college asserts that notification to the coroner, following an assisted death would ensure independent judicial review, which is particularly important given the concerns raised by many individuals, organisations and medical royal colleges about the lack of adequate safeguards in the Bill for vulnerable people.[25]

It is also important to note that **The Royal College of Nursing (RCN)** has a neutral position on the principle of assisted dying.[26] They state, "*this position allows us to represent and support all nursing staff, regardless of their personal or professional stance on assisted dying, while focusing on practical measures to ensure patient safety, workforce protection, and the effective delivery of* high-quality, end-of-life care." They believe nursing staff must have the right to choose whether to be involved or not in assisted dying, in line with the principles of the Nursing and Midwifery Council (NMC) Code. The proposed legislation in England and Wales requires that only a doctor would be permitted to provide the patient with the substance to end their own life. However, in Scotland and the Isle of Man this permission extends to registered nurses.

A view from the Chief Medical Officers

The Chief Medical Officers of the UK, who we have already quoted have set the scene in a cautious and clear way

"This has to be a decision for society as a whole, expressed through Parliament.
Whatever Parliament decides, we believe the medical profession will be unanimous on 2 things:

- *that we must not undermine the provision of good end-of-life care for all including the outstanding work done by palliative care clinicians*

- *that individual doctors and other healthcare workers should be able to exercise freedom of conscience as, for example, happens with abortion care currently*

This will, we are sure, be common ground for all sides of this complex societal decision"[27]

A view from a Palliative Care Consultant who supports the legalisation of AD

Professor Sam Ahmedzai, Professor of Palliative Medicine in Sheffield, UK has articulated the views of the minority of his colleagues in Palliative Medicine and published a paper describing how he moved from opposing to supporting the legalisation of AD.[28]

"I support the move to make doctors' professional organisations neutral about assisted dying. As a consultant in hospice and hospital palliative medicine for 27 years, I have, however, been fervently against changing the law in this respect. I remain sceptical about euthanasia (the deliberate ending of a life by an act performed by another person). But in recent years I have radically moved my position on assisted suicide – when a competent person acknowledged to be dying chooses to take a fatal dose of prescribed medication to end his or her own life.

A major factor in my shift has been professional visits to countries where assisted dying is legal. I spent a week in Oregon for the Commission on Assisted Dying meeting healthcare professionals, hospice volunteers, a high court judge, and patients. I am visiting professor at the University of Amsterdam, where I teach palliative medicine to hospital specialists and GPs. In both places good local palliative care coexists with assisted dying, as confirmed globally in a report by the European Association for Palliative Care. In some real cases of terminal suffering discussed with me in the Netherlands I have sometimes thought that British palliative care would have nothing more to offer – therapeutically or spiritually."

A view from a GP on Primary and Palliative Care

Our contributor Dr Elspeth Aspinall describes here her view working as a GP in Scotland with a leading responsibility for Palliative Care:

"As I career down the stairwell racing against time to fulfil my home visits before my afternoon surgery starts, I almost collide with Fiona, my GP mentor, as she returns from seeing her palliative care patients. "It's heartbreaking" Fiona said of the sorrow faced by the families she had been with

that day. "And yet", she paused: "Looking after my palliative patients is what I come to work for …It is an honour, to walk with these families through their darkest hours and to move heaven and earth to make them feel at peace".

As a new, underconfident and rather anxious GP trainee, I marveled, wide eyed, at Fiona's serenity in the face of such tragic circumstances. At this stage in my career, I was consumed with doubt about my own abilities to have a meaningful impact on patients and families lived experience of death and dying.

Over the coming months, Fiona, and my trainer Paul, supported me to develop my skills and confidence in looking after patients with palliative needs, and to effectively manage their end-of-life care.

4 Months later

I am by the side of a young lady dying from lung cancer. We sat on her sofa. She grips my hand, a terrified look in her eyes. It is Christmas time which only magnifies her desolation. "In the bleak midwinter" is the only bearable festive song that springs to mind. I find myself speaking from the heart as I said: "I will do everything I possibly can to ease your suffering and to enable you to live as well as you can for as long as you can ". From the moment I saw the tight angst in her face and eyes begin to soften, my passion for palliative care was alight.

2025

My "imposter part" finds it inconceivable that I am now a strategic lead for palliative care in Grampian Region. Through this role, I now have a responsibility to promote the best possible palliative and end of life care across the whole system and population. If this was achieved, could we mitigate for the abject misery experienced by those who believe that to end their life is the only way forward?"

One can only imagine the desolation that is antecedent to a human being considering ending their life as the only way to ease their suffering. When considering the Assisted Dying Bill, a pertinent question surely is: How do we in the UK ensure that effective symptom control is available to all? The World Health Organisation (WHO) describes palliative care as:

"…an approach that improves the quality of life of patients and their families' facing problems associated with life- threatening illness, through the prevention and relief of suffering by means of early identification and impeccable assessment and treatment of pain and other problems, physical, psychosocial, and spiritual".[29]

It seems reasonable to surmise that if the UK population had access to adequate and effective palliative and end-of-life care (PEOLC) that the need for assisted dying might be reduced. So, what of our PEOLC services? Johansen et al.[30] in their report "Time to Care, a nationally representative survey of experience at the end of life in England and Wales" found the following:

- fewer than half of those who died had any contact with specialist palliative care – from a hospital or community palliative care team, or hospice
- contact with palliative care was disproportionately low for people without cancer, such as those with heart disease (24%) or dementia (25%)
- almost one in five (19%) people who died had no contact with a GP in their final 3 months of life (either in person or over the telephone)
- only 29% reported contact with palliative care doctors, nurses, or 'hospice at home' teams to help support them at home
- only 19% reported receiving support from a palliative care team when in hospital

- only 10% reported support in a care home
- almost half (49%) reported they were unhappy with one or more aspect(s) of care in the last week of life
- 35% of those who died were reported to be severely or overwhelmingly affected by pain and 40% were severely or overwhelmingly affected by breathlessness

These figures suggest that we have much room to improve our populations access to PEOLC services and perhaps the focus on the assisted dying bill is a distraction from prioritising attaining the best possible PEOLC standards for all our population. Furthermore, Hospice UK, an organisation representing 200 hospices across the UK, has repeatedly promulgated the dire financial straits our hospices find themselves in. To date, most hospice funding arises from charitable donations with around one third from government. It has been intimated that assisted dying would be funded from existing NHS budgets. As a bare minimum it would seem just for funding for assisted dying to be matched with an increase in funding for 24/7 palliative care services.

With access to palliative care services already suboptimal, the proposed assisted dying legislation could make matters worse: it is possible that patients may put barriers to engaging with palliative care services for fear that assisted dying is synonymous with palliative care.

Most palliative care is delivered by primary care multi-disciplinary teams (MDTs), with only a small proportion of all palliative patients requiring specialist palliative medical intervention. General Practitioners (GPs) work closely with community nursing teams to alleviate suffering and ensure that their palliative patients live as well as is possible until the end of life. Primary care teams also work to ensure their patients and loved ones experience a peaceful end of life. This unique role potentially makes GPs the one of the most likely professional groups to be involved in the assisted dying process.

A BMA 2020 survey[31] on assisted dying reported:

Key Findings

*Surveyed members' views on a change in the law to permit doctors to prescribe drugs for eligible patients to **self-administer** to end their own life*

- *Four in ten (40%) surveyed members expressed the view that the British Medical Association (BMA) should actively support attempts to change the law, one in three (33%) favoured opposition and one in five (21%) felt the BMA should adopt a neutral position, neither actively supporting nor actively opposing attempts to change the law to permit doctors to prescribe life-ending drugs.*
- *Half (50%) of surveyed members personally believed that there should be a change in the law to permit doctors to prescribe life-ending drugs. Four in ten (39%) were opposed, with a further one in ten (11%) undecideds.*
- *Forty-five percent of surveyed members were not prepared to actively participate in the process of prescribing life-ending drugs, should it be legalised. Over a third (36%) said they would be prepared to actively participate, and a further two in ten (19%) were undecided on the matter*

*Surveyed members' views on a change in the law to permit doctors to **administer** drugs to end an eligible patient's life*

- *Four in ten (40%) surveyed members expressed the view that the BMA should actively oppose attempts to change the law to permit doctors to administer life-ending drugs. Three in ten (30%) favoured support, and 23% felt the BMA should adopt a neutral stance of neither actively supporting nor actively opposing attempts to change the law.*
- *Forty-six percent of surveyed members personally opposed a change in the law to permit doctors to administer life-ending drugs, with a further 37% supportive and 17% undecided.*
- *Fifty-four percent of surveyed members said that they would not be willing to actively participate in the process of administering life-ending drugs, should it be legalised. A quarter (26%) said they would, and one in five (20%) were undecided on the matter.*

The specialties arguably less likely to be involved in the actual process were more in favour (anaesthetics, emergency medicine, intensive care and obstetrics & gynaecology). The specialties with more tangible involvement with palliative and end of life care (clinical oncology, general practice, geriatric medicine and palliative care) were notably in general less supportive of the proposed legislation. These figures suggest a reluctance of physicians to actively engage in the process of assisted dying.[31]

Can we envisage as the impact on GPs should they have this responsibility without additional resources and capacity? The profession is known to be in crisis with two in five GPs intending to leave the profession in the next 5 years; one third at risk of burnout and seventy per cent reporting their job to be very or extremely stressful.[32–34] It is probable that if the additional responsibility is deemed to reside with GPs without additional resources and capacity, this will increase the threat to the profession's resilience and sustainability.

We will discuss the international experience of AD on patients, caregivers and their families in Chapter 9. Complication rates are low but the process of consultation, decision and delivery of AD and the appropriate aftercare for bereaved loved ones, are demanding and time consuming. The requirement for healthcare professional input to AD inevitably falls on primary care to a substantial extent.

There is deep concern among GPs and others about the potential for moral and psychological injury to both patients, loved ones and GPs. Doctors migrate towards the profession because they hunger to make others' lives better. At the point in time where they can no longer preserve and prolong life, they are driven to ease suffering, promote quality of life and to covet a peaceful death for their patient and loved ones. It follows that the conflict a clinician could feel, in being accountable for ending their patients' lives, could sustain significant trauma, with moral and psychological injury. The impact on the doctor patient relationship must also be considered. This partnership is fundamental to achieving optimal patient outcomes through shared decision making. GPs look after communities and generations of families. There is conceivable vulnerability to the doctor patient relationship should the bereft, in their grief, attribute blame to their GP for their loved one's death.

In applying an ethical framework to the proposed legislation, patient autonomy in choosing to end their life, and the benefit of an absolute end to suffering must be balanced with the potential trauma to patients and loved ones of AD. General Practice is an already vulnerable vocation. Presupposition that GPs will be involved in this process escalates risk to the professions viability and may threaten the doctor patient relationship. Equitable access to effective palliative care in primary care, community hospices and specialist settings may ameliorate the need for our terminally ill patients seeking an assisted death. It would seem just that as a society there is sufficient resources to effective palliative care in parallel with the progression of the assisted dying bill.

Twycross concluded in his review paper,[35] a palatable path from a primary care perspective could be the devolution of assisted dying to a "Department of Assisted Dying". This would be under the jurisdiction of legal professionals and technicians with doctors only responsibility being confirming patient eligibility.

Overall medical professional views

All the healthcare professions and disciplines emphasise the central role of Palliative Care for all patients facing choices at the end of their lives. They all emphasise the vital importance of protecting vulnerable patients and appropriate safeguards. When facing severe pressures on healthcare services, these must not be allowed to reduce the quality of a service for AD.

Surveys of college members reveal that many healthcare professionals reporting are supportive of providing access for their patients to AD although only a smaller minority are willing to provide direct input into the services. Almost without exception healthcare professionals favour the option to allow an opt out of the delivery of AD services while recognising the importance of timely opportunities to provide patients with access to other colleagues to provide the appropriate input.

The vital importance of ready access to well-planned training programmes for professional involved in AD is strongly supported.

For most, the barriers appear to be practical, logistic and resource driven. Practical issues such as funding, training, and assessment of capacity are prominent. Ethical issues less so. Although there is great concern about whether then current legislation is sufficient to protect vulnerable patients or those with mental health issues which may lead to coercion. There is a general concern about the personal, professional and healthcare service impact of the changes in the law on AD among healthcare professionals. Colleagues in palliative medicine are deeply concerned about the impact of AD on their relationship with patients and patterns of service delivery. General practitioners are at the forefront of the work and the logistic and resource pressures. In some countries, the provision of medical assistance in dying is becoming a specialised activity to some extent.

Learning from and utilising expertise from the Royal Colleges and professional Learned Societies should be central to optimising the finer details of any AD legislation to make sure the service is workable, efficient and acceptable to healthcare professional and ultimately will lead to a safer and more patient focused services.

This chapter has demonstrated the intense and caring engagement of healthcare professionals, as organisations and individuals, in the discussions and debates surround AD and its legislation. Many are organisations are neutral but there is no consensus. In Chapters 4–7, we will review the international experience which can help to inform UK views and plans.

References

1. RCP survey results by speciality. Taken from RCP briefing – Assisted Dying 0719.pdf. Available from: https://www.rcplondon.ac.uk/guidelines-policy/rcp-parliamentary-briefing-functioning-existing-law-relating-assisted-dying (accessed 16 July 2025).

2. 2019 assisted dying survey results. No majority view moves RCP position to neutral. Available from: https://rcp.ac.uk/news-and-media/news-and-opinion/2019-assisted-dying-survey-results-no-majority-view-moves-rcp-position-to-neutral (accessed 16 July 2025).

3. The RCP clarifies its position on assisted dying. Available from: https://www.rcp.ac.uk/policy-and-campaigns/policy-documents/rcp-position-statement-on-the-terminally-ill-adults-end-of-life-bill-9th-may-2025/ (Accessed 05/10/2025)

4. RCR responds to progress of the Assisted Dying Bill. Available from: https://www.rcr.ac.uk/news-policy/latest-updates/rcr-responds-to-progress-of-the-assisted-dying-bill (accessed 16 July 2025).

5. Treleaven L, Komesaroff P, La Brooy C, et al. A review of the utility of prognostic tools in predicting 6-month mortality in cancer patients, conducted in the context of voluntary assisted dying. Intern Med J. 2023;53(12):2180–2197.

6. Evenblij K, Pasman HRW, van Delden JJM, et al. Physicians' experiences with euthanasia: a cross-sectional survey amongst a random sample of Dutch physicians to explore their concerns, feelings and pressure. BMC Fam Pract. 2019;20(1):177.

7. Wibisono S, Minto K, Lizzio-Wilson M, et al. Attitudes toward and experience with assisted-death services and psychological implications for health practitioners: a narrative systematic review. Omega (Westport). 2025;91(2):590–612.

8. Winters JP, Jaye C, Pickering NJ, et al. Providing medically assisted dying in Canada: a qualitative study of emotional and moral impact. J Med Ethics. 2025;51(6):400–410.

9. Winters JP, Walker S, Pickering NJ, et al. Conduit or conductor? Physician providers' descriptions of their role as MAiD assessors in the first years after legalisation in Canada. J Med Ethics. 2025:jme-2024-110518.

10. Association for Palliative Medicine Position Statement On Assisted Dying. https://apmonline.org/wp-content/uploads/APM-Position-Statement-on-Assisted-Dying-October-2024-v2.pdf

11. Yon Y, Mikton CR, Gassoumis ZD, et al. Elder abuse prevalence in community settings: a systematic review and meta-analysis. Lancet Glob Health. 2017;5(2):e147–e156.

12. Hitchens. How assisted suicide will undo the NHS. Available from: https://www.compactmag.com/article/how-assisted-suicide-will-destroy-the-nhs (accessed 16 July 2025).

13. Hitchens. The assisted suicide bill should not survive. Available from: https://www.spectator.co.uk/article/the-assisted-suicide-bill-should-not-survive (accessed 16 July 2025).

14. House of Commons Health and Social Care Committee Assisted Dying/Assisted Suicide Second Report of Session 2023–24. Available from: https://committees.parliament.uk/publications/43582/documents/216484/default (accessed 16 July 2025).

15. Better End of Life 2024. Time to care: findings from a nationally representative survey of experiences at the end of life in England and Wales. Available from: https://www.mariecurie.org.uk/document/experiences-at-the-end-of-life-in-england-and-wales (accessed 16 July 2025).

16. Streeting says he changed mind on assisted dying over UK's poor palliative care. Available from: https://www.telegraph.co.uk/politics/2024/10/29/health-secretary-wes-streeting-assisted-dying-nhs-care (accessed 16 July 2025).

17. Jones DA. Evidence of harm: assessing the impact of assisted dying/assisted suicide on palliative care. Available from: https://bioethics.org.uk/media/t1bf0icr/evidence-of-harm-assessing-the-impact-of-assisted-dying-assisted-suicide-on-palliative-care-prof-david-albert-jones.pdf (accessed 16 July 2025).

18. Terminally Ill Adults (End of Life) Bill. Supplementary written evidence submitted by Dr Jamilla Hussain (TIAB252). https://publications.parliament.uk/pa/cm5901/cmpublic/TerminallyIllAdults/memo/TIAB252.htm

19. BMA. Public and professional opinion on physician-assisted dying. Available from: https://www.bma.org.uk/media/ejcdado1/public-and-professional-opinion-on-pad-updated-jan-2025.pdf (accessed 16 July 2025).

20. Briefing from the Royal College of College of Psychiatrists for MPs | The Terminally Ill Adults (End of Life) Bill for England and Wales | Report Stage & Third Reading. 16

May 2025. Available from: https://www.rcpsych.ac.uk/docs/default-source/improving-care/better-mh-policy/policy/assisted-dying-assisted-suicide-january-2025/rcpsych-briefing-the-terminally-ill-adults-(end-of-life)-bill-report-stage-and-third-reading.pdf?sfvrsn=e7bfbf1c_1 (accessed 16 July 2025).

21. RCGP shifts to position of neither supporting nor opposing assisted dying. 14 March 2025. Available from: https://www.rcgp.org.uk/news/rcgp-position-on-assisted-dying (accessed 30 June 2025).

22. Royal College of Surgeons of England. Assisted Dying. 2023. Available from: https://www.rcseng.ac.uk/about-the-rcs/government-relations-and-consultation/position-statements-and-reports/assisted-dying/ (accessed 23 February 2025).

23. Enventure Research. Assisted Dying research: research report. Available from: https://www.rcseng.ac.uk/-/media/Files/RCS/About-rcs/Government-relations-consultation/RCS-England-Assisted-Dying-Survey--Research-Report.pdf (accessed 23 February 2025).

24. Royal College of Anaesthetists Assisted Dying/Suicide Research. November 2024. Available from: https://www.rcoa.ac.uk/sites/default/files/documents/2025-02/RCoA-assisted-dying-assisted-suicide-report-Feb25update.pdf (accessed 16 July 2025).

25. Royal College of Pathologists statement on the Terminally Ill Adults (End of Life) Bill. Available from: https://www.rcpath.org/discover-pathology/news/royal-college-of-pathologists-statement-on-the-terminally-ill-adults-end-of-life-bill.html#:~:text=OK-,Royal%20College%20of%20Pathologists%20statement%20on%20the%20Terminally%20Ill%20Adults,assisted%20death%20has%20taken%20place (accessed 30 June 2025).

26 RCN position on assisted dying in the UK and Crown Dependencies. Available from: https://www.rcn.org.uk/About-us/Our-Influencing-work/Position-statements/rcn-position-on-assisted-dying-in-the-uk-and-crown-dependencies#:~:text=The%20Royal%20College%20of%20Nursing,and%20autonomy%20of%20nursing%20staff (accessed 16 July 2025).

27. UK chief medical officers and NHS England National Medical Director. 2024. Assisted Dying debate: advice to doctors. https://www.gov.uk/government/publications/assisted-dying-bill-debate-advice-to-doctors

28. Ahmadzai SH. My journey from anti to pro assisted dying. BMJ. 2012;345: e4592.

29. World Health Organisation. Palliative Care. https://www.who.int/health-topics/palliative-care

30. Johansson T, Pask, Goodrich J, et al. Time to care: findings from a nationally representative survey of experiences at the end of life in England and Wales. https://pure.qub.ac.uk/en/publications/time-to-care-findings-from-a-nationally-representative-survey-of-

31. BMA Physician Assisted Dying Survey. 2020. https://www.bma.org.uk/media/3367/bma-physician-assisted-dying-survey-report-oct-2020.pdf

32. The Health Foundation. Stressed and overworked. 2023. Available from: https://www.health.org.uk/reports-and-analysis/reports/stressed-and-overworked (accessed 15 August 2025).

33. General Medical Council. The state of medical education and practice in the UK. 2021. Available from: https://www.gmc-uk.org/-/media/documents/somep-2021-full-report_pdf-88509460.pdf (accessed 15 August 25).

34. Royal College of General Practitioners. RCGP warns of "mass exodus" if retention of GPs isn't prioritised. 2024. Available from: https://www.rcgp.org.uk/News/mass-exodus-retention-gps-prioritised (accessed 15 August 2025).

35. Twycross R. Assisted Dying: principles, possibilities and practicalities. An English physician's perspective BMC Palliative Care. 2024;23:99.

Chapter 4: International Assisted Dying Laws and Practice: Introduction, Europe and the USA

The British Medical Journal in 2024 has summarised and mapped an updated picture of AD laws around the world.[1] Key points are:

- Legislation to permit AD based on intolerable suffering is in place in Canada, Spain, Portugal, Luxembourg, Belgium, the Netherlands, Austria and Switzerland.

- Legislation to permit AD based on established terminal illness usually with a specified period of life expectancy of 6 or 12 months, is in place in the United States, (Washington, Oregon, Hawaii, California, Colorado, New Mexico, Maine, Vermont, New Jersey and the District of Columbia), Australia (South Australia, Western Australia, Queensland, Victoria, Tasmania, NSW) and in New Zealand.

- There is partially permissive legislation in Columbia, Montana, Germany and Italy.

Heidinger et al.[2] have recently brought together the publicly available international experience of AD from 20 jurisdictions from 1999 to 2023. Canada, Luxembourg, Belgium, the Netherlands, Switzerland, United States, (Washington, Oregon, Hawaii, California, Colorado, Maine, Vermont, New Jersey and the District of Columbia), Australia (South Australia, Western Australia, Queensland, Victoria, Tasmania) and in New Zealand. Ten of these permit Physician Assisted Suicide (PAS where healthcare professionals can provide approved medication to people and supervise self-administration); 15 of the jurisdictions required an estimate of life expectancy to indicate terminal illness, commonly less than 6 or 12 months. In 2023, 282 million people live in countries/legal jurisdictions which permit AD.[2]

They analysed the data for 184,695 AD deaths over the whole period 1999–2023 during which there were a total of 12,933,459 deaths, and AD and total deaths from the most recently reported time estimating the proportion of deaths where AD was involved and the disease types and nature of the AD schemes in each jurisdiction. In the most recently reported time periods, the average proportion of deaths (33,088 AD deaths in 1,675,961 total deaths) was 2%. They range from 0.1% in New Jersey and Washington DC to 4.3% in Canada and 5.1% in The Netherlands. The authors note that some jurisdictions have only recently introduced new laws and schemes, and the rates may still increase. However, in the USA where AD laws were in general introduced in the last decade, the rates are still below 1% in all States included.

Over all the jurisdictions, cancer and Motor Neurone Disease account for about 75% of AD deaths, while they account for about 30% of overall deaths. The diagnoses in AD deaths were cancer (66.5%), nervous system disease (8.1%), circulatory system disease (6.8%), respiratory system disease (4.9%). AD was provided in 16.8% of all deaths from Motor Neurone Disease and 3.7% of all deaths from cancer.

Jurisdictions that permitted only PAS and those that required an estimate of life expectancy had significantly, approximately, two-fold, lower rates of AD as a proportion of all deaths, than those that permitted euthanasia (healthcare professionals could administer medications) or required no estimate of life expectancy.

They were able to comment on the factors which appeared to influence the uptake of AD. Diagnosis (cancer and motor neurone disease) was the most powerful predictor. The eligibility criteria and methods allowed for AD were also influential (see above) but socioeconomic factors and palliative care service availability were not as influential.[3–7] The Journal of the American Medical Association editorial team[8] added a USA perspective, noting that AD has emerged as an option to address the issues of symptom relief and distress at the end of life and calling for the International Classification of Diseases to code for AD to allow global surveillance.[8,9]

Recent Legal Changes in Western Europe

In 2023, Van Bulck et al.[10] summarised changes in medically AD legislation in Western Europe over the previous 5 years. Belgium has made some minor changes to its legislation to alter the duration of validity for advanced directives for euthanasia for people who are in an incurable coma; the process for managing requests for euthanasia that are declined by doctors were streamlined. Luxembourg amended its law to clarify that euthanasia or assisted suicide would be considered a natural death for insurance reasons. In the Netherlands, discussions in Parliament have addressed the question of AD for people who feel that their lives have been long enough and have no meaning ("fulfilled life").

Spain

In Spain, a new law was introduced in June 2021 to allow adult patients with serious or incurable disease or a chronic and incapacitating condition to request that their life be ended. Both the direct administration of a substance or medically assisted suicide prescribed by a medical professional were permitted. Spain was the first Southern European country to legalise AD. The criteria are a severe, chronic, debilitating, or incurable disease, mental competence, the provision of clear information, four separate requests, supportive medical reports, and an evaluating committee before a final consent. Additional safeguards include a regional commission of seven people including healthcare experts with strict timelines. Healthcare workers can opt out and patients can change their minds or delay the decision. The Catholic Church strongly opposes euthanasia. Initial reports suggest a lower rate of uptake of the choice for AD in Spain compared to Canada and New Zealand, with most patients opting for euthanasia rather than assisted suicide. Neurological conditions were initially the largest number of diagnoses, more than cancer which is the largest group in Canada and New Zealand.[11,12]

Espericueta[13] summarised the experience from June 2021 to December 2023. There were 1515 requests and 697 people accessed AD. The uptake of AD increased from 0.01% of deaths in 2021 to 0.07% in 2023, well below international figures. Waiting time from request was 67 days in 2023 and has fallen since the system was introduced. Most (96%) of people chose intravenous administration of medication. By 2023, the most frequent diagnosis was cancer. There remain controversies and legal challenges around the eligibility of those with mental illnesses, euthanasia in prison, advance directives and the degree of conscientious objection of healthcare professionals[13] with active research into professional attitudes.[14,15]

France

In France, the development of legislation to permit AD has been complex and challenging.[16–19] A bill to legalise assisted suicide was proposed in 2021 but did not progress. A brisk public and political debate ensued. French public opinion was reported to support the introduction of AD with approximately 70% of those consulted supporting the widening of end-of-life choices. In April 2024, the French Government proposed a bill to take to Parliament which had provision for AD for competent adults with incurable disease and a short to medium expected lifetime, together with physical and psychological pain which was resistant to treatment and could not be tolerated. In parallel the Government announced a 10-year package to strengthen palliative care throughout France, committing to spend over one billion euros in that time. Disruptions to French parliamentary politics delayed progress with the legislation.

In 2025,[20,21] however, the French National Assembly approved a Bill legalising AD by 305 votes to 199. The Bill proceeds to the Senate and a second reading in the National Assembly, possibly becoming law in 2027. A bill for a right to palliative care was also supported. The current Bill which will like face amendment identifies

- a serious and incurable disease
- life-threatening and in its advanced or terminal phases
- psychiatric diseases and dementia are not eligible
- constant physical or psychological suffering
- a patient's must freely manifest his or her intention
- wait 48 hours and then confirm it
- the lethal medication would be self-administered by the patient; or by a medical assistant if the patient were incapable
- authorisation a doctor, but only after consultation with other doctors
- medical staff who oppose assisted dying would not have to carry it out

There were strong religious and some professional objections especially from the Palliative Care discipline to the Bill and its passage through the Senate may be controversial.[21–23]

Germany and Austria

In Germany, in 2020 a pre-existing ban on assisted suicide services was ruled to be in breach of the Constitution[24] and new laws to regulate AD are under consideration.[25] AD is legal in Germany under certain circumstances. The Constitutional Court text reads *"The right to a self-determined death includes the freedom to take one's own life. Where an individual decides to end their own life, having reached this decision based on how they personally define quality of life and a meaningful existence, their decision must, in principle, be respected by state and society as an act of personal autonomy and self-determination. The freedom to take one's own life also encompasses the freedom to seek and, if offered, make use of assistance provided by third parties for this purpose".* Healthcare prescribers can provide drugs to patients. Close relatives of the patients may assist patients. However, physically ending a patient's life, is still illegal. Germany is still debating how to legally regulate euthanasia.

Farr et al.[26] give a summary of the current complexities. The ban on physicians assisting patient in AD has been removed from the German Medical Code of Conduct at a National level and some Regional (Lander) Codes have been amended to match. The German Medical Association do not regard AD as a genuinely medical task. Just over half of German Oncologists report being asked about AD in 2023,[27,28] GP's only "occasionally".[26]

In Austria, AD under strict regulation was legalised in 2022.[29,30] In Austria, AD is restricted to people with a serious, incurable illness. The Statute on the "Will to Die" requires

- Limited to individuals with a severe, permanent illness affecting their entire life. Minors are excluded.
- There must be no doubt that the person is capable of making a decision.
- A mental health assessment (psychiatrist/psychologist) is required if there is a suspicion of pathological mental impairment.
- A waiting period of 12 weeks is mandated to address acute and distressing symptoms and treatable crises. For those in the terminal phase of an illness, this period is reduced to 2 weeks.
- A valid patient's dying will allow individuals to obtain a lethal preparation from a pharmacy.
- The medical consultations to evaluate the request must include a doctor with a qualification in Palliative medicine.

In 2022, 57 people claimed AD in Austria.[30] There may be difficulties in accessing AD in Austrian healthcare institutions.[31] **The ASCIRS** platform is a reporting and learning system of the Austrian Palliative Care Society. It is intended to contribute to learning about the practice of assisted suicide in Austria and to learn from the observations and experiences of those involved.[32]

Ireland

In Ireland, in 2020 a bill referred to as "dying with dignity" was introduced and initially supported. A Joint Committee on AD was established and in its Final Report in March 2024 it said, "*The Committee recommends that the Government introduces legislation allowing for assisted dying, in certain restricted circumstances as set out in the recommendations in this report*".[33] In October 2024, a majority of members of the Dail voted to note the report but there are many further steps before such legislation could be enacted.[34]

Italy

In Italy, AD may be permitted under some circumstances.[35,36] Riva[36] noted "*Although in Italy there is currently no effective law on physician-assisted suicide or euthanasia, Decision No 242 issued by the Italian Constitutional Court on September 25, 2019, established that an individual who, under specific circumstances, has facilitated the implementation of an independent and freely formed resolve to commit suicide by another individual is exempt from criminal liability*". There have been requests for assisted suicide generating uncertainty. The Tuscan regional government has passed a law permitting AD but it may face challenges for the national government.[37]

Portugal

Portugal's Parliament approved in 2023 a law permitting assistance with dying for patients who are terminally ill with severe symptoms. The law applies to mentally competent adults (18+) who are terminally ill or suffering from a serious and incurable illness or injury, and experiencing intense, lasting, and unbearable suffering.[38,39] The law is not yet in force and faces legal and regulatory challenges.[38–40]

Belgium

Lewis discussed the experience of AD in Belgium to 2020.[41] Belgium legalized euthanasia in 2002, allowing competent adults in a medically hopeless condition who are suffering unbearably from a serious disorder without remedy to request euthanasia, provided it is voluntary, in writing, and approved by independent physicians. In 2014, the law was extended to minors, involving only a few cases. The Federal Commission for the Control and Evaluation of Euthanasia ensures compliance and transparency. More recently, the long-term experience from 2002 to 2023 has given Wels and Hamarat[42] the opportunity to examine long term trends in substantial number (33,647) of patients. Euthanasia increased from 236 cases in 2003 to 2700 cases in 2021, 2.4% of all deaths. Most (65%) of diagnoses were cancer with 15% reporting multimorbidity. In 85% of cases death was expected within 1 year. Most (73%) of patients reported both physical and mental suffering.

In the first decade, up to 2015, the rate of increase was steep, as the new regulations were taken up. From 2015, it slowed, and changes thereafter were largely explained by demographic changes (the ageing population) although there was also some evening out of cases across the country and between the genders. Multimorbidity was an increasing feature of the diagnoses reported. Cases involving dementia and psychiatric disorders were stable in numbers. They confirm Lewis's observations[41] that practitioners were compliant with the regulations and eligibility criteria.[42]

Despite the reassuring statistics from the Belgium data, in depth interviews with Belgium health professionals in 2025[43] still report considerable pressure and stress in the delivery of AD. Challenges were reported from the framing of the law, workload pressures; clashing views about euthanasia and the processes around AD are still not always well understood.[43]

The Netherlands

In the Netherlands, AD became permitted under regulations in 2002 through the legislation "Termination of Life on Request and Assisted Suicide (Review Procedures) Act". The Netherlands is often quoted as the jurisdiction with the most widely permissive AD legislation. The Netherlands Government website[44] gives the details:

"Difference between termination of life on request and assisted suicide

- *Termination of life on request is when a physician administers the substances to the patient.*
- *Assisted suicide is when the physician hands a lethal substance to the patient who then ingests it.*

Below, the word 'euthanasia' is used to refer to both forms of helping a person to die.
Only the patient can request euthanasia.

The patient must make the request personally. A request for euthanasia made by another person on behalf of the patient cannot be granted. It must always be clear that the request has been made by the patient personally.

The request must have been made without any undue influence from others. The physician must be satisfied that the patient's request is voluntary and well considered.

Euthanasia and minors

A child may request euthanasia from the age of 12. However, the following additional requirements apply:

- *the child must be capable of assessing and understanding what is best for them in their situation.*
- *if a child is aged 12–15, euthanasia can only be carried out with the consent of the child's parent or parents, or the child's guardian.*
- *if a child is aged 16 or 17, the parent(s) or guardian must be consulted in the decision-making process, but their consent is not required.*

Oral request for euthanasia

It is not necessary for a patient to make a euthanasia request in writing. An oral request is sufficient.

Advance directive

A patient who is decisionally competent can draw up a written request for euthanasia, an 'advance directive'. An advance directive can replace an oral request for euthanasia if at a later point the patient is no longer able to express their will with regard to euthanasia (due to, for instance, advanced dementia or reduced consciousness).

It is important that the patient describe as specifically as possible the circumstances in which they would wish their life to be terminated. It is the responsibility of the patient to discuss their advance directive with the physician when drafting or updating the document. The physician should include this information in the patient's medical records.

There is no prescribed format for an advance directive, and the patient can write in their own words.

Due care criteria

According to the Termination of Life on Request and Assisted Suicide (Review Procedures) Act the physician must:

1. *be satisfied that the patient's **request is voluntary and well considered**.*
2. *be satisfied that the patient's **suffering is unbearable, with no prospect of improvement**.*
3. *have **informed** the patient about their **situation and their prognosis**.*
4. *have come to the conclusion, together with the patient, that there is **no reasonable alternative** in the patient's situation.*
5. *have **consulted** at least one other, **independent physician**, who must see the patient and give a written opinion on whether the due care criteria set out in (1) to (4) have been fulfilled; and*
6. *have exercised **due medical care and attention** in terminating the patient's life or assisting in the patient's suicide.*

Under what conditions is euthanasia allowed?

Euthanasia is only allowed for patients whose unbearable suffering with no prospect of improvement has a medical dimension. This can be the case with somatic diseases such as cancer or cardiovascular disease, but also with psychiatric disorders, dementia or multiple geriatric syndromes. The Act does not allow euthanasia in cases where a person is 'finished with life' or deems their life to be 'completed'.

Patient has no right to euthanasia and physician is not obliged to perform euthanasia. Physicians are not obliged to grant a request for euthanasia, even if the due care criteria set out in the Act have been fulfilled. Patients do not have a right to euthanasia, and physicians are entitled to refuse to carry out euthanasia, for instance because of their religious beliefs.

If a physician is unwilling to perform euthanasia, it is prudent from a medical professional point of view to inform the patient accordingly as early as possible. The patient can then, if they so wish, contact another physician. Physicians may also refer the patient to a colleague.

Notification and review

A physician who has performed euthanasia must always notify this to the municipal pathologist, providing a detailed report. The municipal pathologist investigates the death and must then send the notification, including all the associated documents, to one of the five regional euthanasia review committees in the Netherlands. This committee reviews the reports and the euthanasia procedure and establishes whether the physician satisfied all the due care criteria in performing euthanasia.

If the committee finds that the physician failed to fulfil one or more due care criteria, it is legally required to report its findings to the Public Prosecution Service (OM) and the Health and Youth Care Inspectorate (IGJ). These bodies then consider what further steps need to be taken. For instance, they can file a disciplinary complaint against the physician or decide to prosecute the physician. A physician who is found guilty of unlawfully performing euthanasia is liable to:

- in the case of termination of life on request: up to 12 years in prison, or a fine.
- in the case of assisted suicide: up to 3 years in prison, or a fine.

The 2024 report of the Regional Euthanasia Review Committees in the Netherlands[45] highlighted

"In 2024, the Regional Euthanasia Review Committees (RTE) received 9,958 reports of euthanasia. This is 10% more than in 2023. The number of euthanasia reports relative to the total mortality rate increased from 5.4% to 5.8%.

Euthanasia reports (86.29%) involved common physical conditions such as cancer, nervous system disorders, lung diseases, and/or cardiovascular diseases. In 427 reports, euthanasia was performed on a patient with a form of dementia. In 219 reports, the suffering stemmed (largely) from one or more mental health conditions. The RTE received 397 reports concerning people with a combination of age-related conditions. Finally, there were 232 reports in the residual category "other conditions.

In six cases, the RTE concluded that the physician had not met the due care requirements when performing euthanasia. Two of these reports involved the failure to (properly) consult a consultant. One report concerned the extreme caution a physician must exercise when the euthanasia request stems (largely) from suffering resulting from a mental illness. In the other three reports, the Guidelines for Performing Euthanasia had not been followed in a complicated procedure".[46]

Schweren et al.[47] studied the small but increasing group of **young Dutch people** who requested AD based on **psychiatric suffering** between 2012 and 2021. There were 397 applications by 353 individuals (73% female, mean age 21 years), increasing from 10 in 2012 to 39 in 2021. 188 were retracted; 178 were rejected. 12 people died through AD. Seventeen people died by suicide during the application process. Those who died had long treatment histories and prominent suicidality.[47] Schweren et al. emphasise the need for more prospective research to understand the psychiatric issues and treatment needs of this group.

Campbell et al.[48,49] investigated AD for **mature minors** in the Netherlands and Belgium and its relevance to the ongoing debate in Canada. Cases are rare with only three cases in Belgium between 2016 and 2018 and a total of 16 cases in the Netherlands between 2002 and 2020. The reported rationale was usually intolerable suffering and hopeless care situations. Approaches are different with the Netherlands having formal are limits (see above) and Belgium requiring the patient to be judged to have the capacity for discernment.

AD on psychiatric grounds is permitted in the Netherlands and Belgium with differences between the regulation between the two (see Ref. 50). Verhofstadt et al.[50] reported on the numbers involved and the ethical and clinical debates. Between 2002 and 2023, there were 457 cases of AD on psychiatric grounds in Belgium and about 900 in the Netherlands, less than 1.5% of all AD cases. The proportion of rejected requests is higher than in cases of physical diagnoses. They discuss the trends and factors influencing requests and the assessment. The influence of media representation of AD on young people is highlighted. Psychiatric service pressures and reluctance of psychiatrists to engage in assessments are sources of concern.

Dutch regulations for AD do not require that **relatives** of people making requests are involved, but most doctors (80%) want to know relatives' opinions and they are influential but not decisive.[51]

Dutch ethicists play centrals roles in the national and international debates around AD, may be electively involved in consideration of requests and are formally represented on the Dutch Euthanasia Regional Review Committees.[52–55] Following parliamentary proposals in 2016, consideration has been given to AD for individuals over the age of 75 years who feel their lives are complete. An individual's right to autonomy has been a feature of the proposals; the risk of inappropriate uptake of the option influenced by mental health concerns or societal pressures and its impact on a stable and functioning system have been features opposing arguments.[53,54] The issue is divisive and unlikely to progress in the foreseeable future.

Luxembourg

Luxembourg passed the "Law on the Right to Die with Dignity" in 2008 after a vote in Parliament and constitutional debates, and it became effective in 2009. The Act is like that in Belgium. The National Commission for Control and Evaluation publishes 2-yearly reports with 34 cases in 2022, a 42% increase from 2021.[56]

The patient's request must be voluntary and made with an understanding of their situation, and they must be mentally competent. 16- to 18-year-olds may also request euthanasia with parents' or guardian's consent. Doctors must seek the opinion of a second doctor. All cases are reviewed by a monitoring commission. The patient must be experiencing unbearable physical or psychological suffering due to an incurable illness. There is no requirement for a diagnosis of a terminal illness or estimation of life expectancy.

The United States experience

Many of the changes in US law and practice which permit AD happened prior to our Workshop and Publication in 2020 and were discussed by Lewis.[41] AD is often referred to as physician-assisted suicide (PAS) in the USA and is legal in eleven US States. It was legalized by a public vote for the 1994 Oregon Death with Dignity Act, but delayed until 1997. In Montana, the route to legalisation was through a judgement by the Montana Supreme Court which ruled in 2009 that state law did not prohibit physician-assisted dying. It was legalized by Washington in 2008, Vermont in 2013, California, Washington, D.C., and Colorado in 2016, Hawaii in 2018, New Jersey in 2019, Maine in 2020, and New Mexico in 2021.

Oregon. The Oregon Act was brought forward by the Oregon Right to Die Political Action Committee. The proposal was that terminally ill patients with less than 6 months life expectancy could receive a prescription for lethal drugs. Approximately two-thirds of patients who receive prescriptions for lethal drugs subsequently take them. Oregon requires a physician to prescribe drugs, and they must be self-administered. In order to be eligible, the patient must be diagnosed by an attending physician as well as by a consulting physician, with a terminal illness that will cause the death of the individual within 6 months. The law states that, in order to participate, a patient must be: (a) 18 years of age or older, (b) a resident of Oregon*, (c) capable of making and communicating health care decisions for him/herself, and (d) diagnosed with a terminal illness that will lead to death within 6 months. It is up to the attending physician to determine whether these criteria have been met. It is required that the patient orally requests the medication at least twice and contributes at least one written request. The physician must notify the patient of alternatives, such as palliative care, hospice and pain management. Lastly the physician is to request but not require the patient to notify their next of kin that they are requesting a prescription for a lethal dose of medication. Assuming all guidelines are met, and the patient is deemed competent and completely sure they wish to end their life, the physician will prescribe the drugs.

In 2022, the Oregon Supreme Court ruled that it was unconstitutional to deny the right to die to individuals from other states who are willing to travel to Oregon to use the law.

Montana. Aid in dying is legal in Montana through a state supreme court decision. Montana Supreme Court ruled that state law allows for terminally ill Montanans to request lethal medication from a physician under existing statutes, in 2009.

Vermont. In May 2013, the Vermont Legislature passed the Patient Choice and Control at End of Life Act based on the Oregon model, the first state to pass an assisted death law through legislative process. Vermont residents 18 years old or older who are mentally capable adults with a terminal illness and a prognosis of 6 months or less to live can make an oral request and obtain a lethal dose of medication from a physician to hasten their death.

California. The California legislature passed the California End of Life Option Act, a bill legalising the practice in September 2015 The bill allows medication to be prescribed by a licensed physician to a patient who is over the age of 18, living with a chronic and life altering condition that is irreversible, and must be of sound mind to make these decisions.

Colorado. In 2016, Colorado voters passed through the ballot process, the Colorado End of Life Options Act, making assisted death legal among patients with a terminal illness.

District of Columbia. The Death with Dignity Act of 2015 went into effect in 2017.

Hawaii. Since 2019, Hawaii has legally allowed AD, based on the Oregon and Washington state models.

Maine. The Maine Death with Dignity Act was introduced in the state legislature and signed into law in 2019.

New Jersey. The Aid in Dying for the Terminally Ill Act was passed by the State Assembly and went into effect in 2019.

New Mexico. In 2021, the Elizabeth Whitefield End-of-Life Options Act became law and took effect after the bill passed the New Mexico Legislature, legalising assisted suicide in the state.

Washington. Washington voters approved the Death with Dignity Act by general election in 2008 Washington›s rules and restrictions are similar to Oregon›s.

In 2022, Kozlov et al. aggregated the basic data on the uptake of AD across the USA from nine jurisdictions.[57] They noted that 74 million people in the USA live in a jurisdiction that permits AD and that there are ongoing discussions on the legislative agenda in 14 additional states. Their study records

- 8451 prescriptions for AD and 5329 deaths
- More men than women accessed AD (53% vs. 47%)
- Most people accessing AD were non-Hispanic white individuals (96%)
- Median age of AD deaths was 74 years
- 72% had some college education
- 74% had cancer and 10% had a neurological condition
- 88% informed their families
- 87% were enrolled in hospice or palliative care
- 90% died at home

In all the jurisdictions reported there was an increase in the proportion of AD compared to all deaths between 1998 and 2020 but in no case did the proportion exceed 1%.[57]

Grubbs et al.[58] conducted a rapid systematic review of publications from the USA 2019–2024, collecting regulatory and legal issues, healthcare professionals experience, patient and caregiver experience and disparate access issues. They note

- Current American Medical Association guidelines allow physicians to follow their consciences in jurisdictions where AD is legal.
- The National Hospice and Palliative Care Organisation supports the individual's right to choose AD where it is legal.
- Nurses are not allowed to give AD medications but are allowed to care for patients undergoing AD. Conscientious objections are allowed.
- Oregon and Vermont do not require state residency.

They identified 10 articles addressing the Healthcare Professionals experience reporting that some 26% of doctors felt conflicted about AD consultations and delivery while 76% reported fulfilment in their recent AD experience. Most nurses reported being comfortable with the AD process. Religious convictions reduce the proportion of HCPs who supported AD. Reports from Oregon and Washington recorded complications in the patient experience of AD in 4% of cases. No State funded insurance covers the cost of AD and most commercial insurance does not do so and the cost of prescriptions in the USA is rising to about $700. The statistics reflect this with more wealthy and educated Americans accessing AD.

Relatively little is known about the identity and experience of the clinicians who provide AD in the USA and elsewhere. There are some trends towards specialisation with a relatively small group of clinicians undertaking a relatively large proportion of the AD consultations and prescriptions. Pottash et al.[59] surveyed clinicians registered with the American Academy on Medical Aid in Dying and received 72 responses. Most were White; 50% were over 60 years of age and 47% had been in practice for more than 20 years. They were often from Primary care (33%) or Palliative care (25%) and 22% described their practice as a specialised "aid in dying" practice. While many reported having felt conflicted before they undertook any work in AD, after being in the practice they felt no professional or moral conflicts and most felt that the AD legislation balanced access with protection of patients. Harrawood[60] drew attention to the growing role of nurse practitioners in AD practice.

Regnard et al.[61] looked at the changes that have occurred during the 25 years of AD in Oregon. They noted there, as in other jurisdictions,[57] that there had been an increase in cases, from 16 in 1998 to 278 in 2022. Despite an increase in the proportion of patients drawing on government funding, financial pressures were still noted by people accessing AD. The data allowed an assessment of the duration of the clinical relationship between the patient and the doctor to whom the AD requests were made, and it had decreased considerably from 18 weeks in 2010 to 5 weeks in 2022.

Disabled people who cannot self-administer medications have limited access to AD in the USA. The requirement for an estimated life expectancy of less than 6 months presents especial challenges to patients in the USA with some neurodegenerative conditions.[58] Kious[62] notes that patients with neurodegenerative conditions may not be able to make the necessary verbal or written requests or self-administer medication within the required 6-month time frame for life expectancy which may limit their access to AD.

Macmillan et al.[63] evaluated data on the pharmacology of AD in the USA comparing results with one sedative and 3 sedative/cardiotoxin combinations in 3332 reports from 2009 to 2023.

Median time to death was 0.4 hours for the sedative only medication but with some very long duration "outliers" which could be days long. Two sedative/cardiotoxin combinations had median times of 0.8 hours but importantly from 2018 to 2023, with these regimens, the frequency of longer deaths was much reduced.

The Centre to Advance Palliative Care (CAPC) is a US wide organisation which was established in 1999 and gives as its purpose "*to improve the care of people living with serious illness, and their families. For two decades, CAPC has led the nation's growth in sustainable, high-quality palliative care programs and the standardisation of best practice, the process of which aims to rapidly facilitate the translation of a growing body of evidence to implementation in the real world of clinical practice. Today, CAPC also extends its reach beyond palliative care, so that all clinicians treating serious illness have basic palliative care knowledge and skill*".[64] It is funded through membership and philanthropy. CAPC conducts an annual Scorecard review of Palliative Care Services in the USA.[65] The Serious Illness Scorecard assesses from publicly available information

- *Availability of specialty palliative care teams and professionals*
- *Payment for specialty palliative care services*
- *Structures to support awareness and advocacy*
- *Broad clinical education targeted to the care of people with serious illness*
- *Strong structures to meet functional and caregiver support needs*

Each State is given a Score reflecting the CAPC evaluation of its Palliative Care on the Scorecard. The eight highest scores in 2024 were awarded at 4.5 to *Oregon* and Massachusetts, and at 4.0 to *California, New Jersey,* Connecticut, Maryland, Ohio and Illinois (italics indicate States permitting AD). The lowest eight scores at 2.0 or less were given to no States which permit AD. CAPC points out the need for improved Palliative Care across the USA and especially increased workforce. This study does not show that States which permit AD have poorer Palliative Care services. For those who are concerned that introducing AD may harm Palliative Care, it is reassuring that Oregon is scored as having among the best Palliative Care services in the USA

The overall experience of the introduction of AD in Europe and the USA does show that a great deal has been learned and stable working systems have been established. The different criteria for eligibility determine the uptake and experience of patients.

The longer-established European jurisdictions in the Netherlands, Belgium and Luxembourg which permits AD, have eligibility criteria which permit AD for patients who are experiencing "intolerable suffering without a terminal diagnosis or an estimated life expectancy". Some include that such suffering may result from solely mental illness and some include mature minors. These are very different from the proposed eligibility criteria for the UK. Despite these fundamental differences, there are things we can learn from their experience, perhaps especially from the long-term experience of the Benelux countries. Trajectories for the increase in the uptake of access to AD are long and stretch over 10 years before they settle into a stable pattern. Even with mature systems, healthcare professionals can still report workload pressures and stress. Careful monitoring of cases and training of staff are essential. However, AD in these European jurisdictions became, over time, a settled and stable feature of choices at the end of life.

In the USA, criteria for eligibility for AD are much closer to the UK proposals. Established Terminal Illness and an estimated life expectancy are required, and self-administration of medications is usual. The data show lower uptake of AD with these criteria. Some States in the USA have the longest experience of AD choices which are similar to those proposed for the UK. Stable uptake rates and low uptake rates when compared to international averages are seen across all of the permissive US jurisdictions. A wide range of healthcare disciplines and professions are involved. Access to AD is taken to a relatively greater degree by people with socioeconomic and educational advantages and by white people. When assessed by the CAPC with a uniform scoring system, there is no evidence of an association between low scores for the quality of Palliative Care and the States which permit AD.

References

1. Looi MK. Assisted dying laws around the world. BMJ. 2024;387:q2385.

2. Heidinger B, Webber C, Chambaere K, et al. International comparison of underlying disease among recipients of medical assistance in dying. JAMA Intern Med. 2025;185(2):235–237.

3. Mroz S, Dierickx S, Deliens L, et al. Assisted dying around the world: a status questionnaire. Ann Palliat Med. 2021;10(3):3540–3553.

4. Downar J, Fowler RA, Halko R, et al. Early experience with medical assistance in dying in Ontario, Canada: a cohort study. CMAJ. 2020;192(8):E173–E181.

5. Redelmeier DA, Ng K, Thiruchelvam D, et al. Association of socioeconomic status with medical assistance in dying: a case-control analysis. BMJ Open. 2021;11:e043547.

6. Steck N, Junker C, Zwahlen M; Swiss National Cohort. Increase in assisted suicide in Switzerland: did the socioeconomic predictors change? Results from the Swiss National Cohort. BMJ Open. 2018;8(4):e020992.

7. Gerson SM, Koksvik GH, Richards N, et al. The relationship of palliative care with assisted dying where assisted dying is lawful: a systematic scoping review of the literature. J Pain Symptom Manage. 2020;59(6):1287–1303.e1.

8. Stall NM, Gross CP. Centring patients and evidence in debates about medical assistance in dying. JAMA Intern Med. 2025;185;(2):237–238.

9. Güth U, Weitkunat R, McMillan S, et al. When the cause of death does not exist time for the WHO to close the ICD classification gap for medical aid in dying. E Clin Med. 2023;65:102301.

10. Van Bulck L, Quenot JP, Seronde MF, et al. Medically assisted dying in Western Europe: legislation review – what has changed in 5 years? BMJ Support Palliat Care. 2023;13(3): 305–308.

11. Espericueta L. First official report on euthanasia in Spain: a comparison with the Canadian and New Zealand experiences. Med Clin (Barc). 2023;161(10):445–447.

12. Essential guide to assisted suicide in Spain. https://euroweeklynews.com/2024/07/26/essential-guide-to-assisted-suicide-in-spain

13. Espericueta L. Three years of assisted dying in Spain: data, controversies and challenges. Med Clin (Barc). 2025;165(3):107037.

14. Parra Jounou I, Triviño-Caballero R, Cruz-Piqueras M. For, against, and beyond: healthcare professionals' positions on Medical Assistance in Dying in Spain. BMC Med Ethics. 2024;25(1):69

15. Lerma-García D, Parra-Fernández ML, Romero-Blanco C, et al. Nurses' opinions on euthanasia in Spain: an evaluation using a new version of the EAS. BMC Nurs. 2024;23(1):517.

16. Casassus B. French government gives go-ahead to voluntary assisted dying. BMJ. 2024;385:q849.

17. Devi S. Proposed bill to support assisted dying in France. Lancet Oncol. 2024;25(5):e182.

18. Pradat PF, Piazza S, Fourcade C. Letter to the editor: evidence before action: the essential search for evidence-based principles in France's Assisted Dying Legislation. J Palliat Med. 2024;27(4):445–446.

19. Salas S, Economos G, Hugues D, et al. A. Legalisation of euthanasia and assisted suicide: advanced cancer patient opinions – cross-sectional multicentre study. BMJ Support Palliat Care. 2024;13(e3):e1335–e1341.

20. French MPs back law to allow assisted dying. https://www.bbc.co.uk/news/articles/cy8dvgg9wn2o

21. French lawmakers approve assisted dying bill. https://www.lemonde.fr/en/france/article/2025/05/27/french-lawmakers-approve-assisted-dying-bill_6741744_7.html

22. Killing me softly? France's assisted dying bill runs into trouble. https://www.euractiv.com/section/health-consumers/news/killing-me-softly-frances-assisted-dying-bill-runs-into-trouble

23. Economos G, Moulin P, Perceau-Chambard É, et al. for the Société Française d'accompagnement et de Soins Palliatifs (SFAP). Legalised active assistance in dying: palliative care stakeholders' national e-consultation. BMJ Support Palliat Care. 2023:spcare-2022-004081.

24. Judgment of 26 February 2020. https://www.bundesverfassungsgericht.de/SharedDocs/Entscheidungen/EN/2020/02/rs20200226_2bvr234715en.html

25. Wiesing U. The Judgment of the German Federal Constitutional Court regarding assisted suicide: a template for pluralistic states? J Med Ethics. 2022;48:542–546.

26. Farr L, Poeck J, Bozzaro C, et al. Requests for physician-assisted suicide in German general practice: frequency, content, and motives- a qualitative analysis of GPs' experiences. BMC Prim Care. 2025;26(1):122.

27. Schildmann J, Junghanss C, Oldenburg M, et al. Role and responsibility of oncologists in assisted suicide. Practice and views among members of the German Society of Haematology and Medical Oncology. ESMO Open. 2021;6(6):100329.

28. Schildmann J, Cinci M, Kupsch L, et al. Evaluating requests for physician-assisted suicide. A survey among German oncologists. Cancer Med. 2023;12(2):1813–1820.

29. New law allowing assisted suicide takes effect in Austria. https://www.bbc.co.uk/news/world-europe-59847371

30. Masel EK. Perspective: legal, ethical, and medical perspectives of the landscape of assisted suicide in Austria. Wien Klin Wochenschr. 2024;136(13–14):380–381.

31. Kitta A, Ecker F, Zeilinger EL, et al. Statements of Austrian hospices and palliative care units after the implementation of the law on assisted suicide: a qualitative study of web-based publications. Wien Klin Wochenschr. 2024;136(13–14):382–389.

32. The ASCIRS platform: a reporting and learning system of the Austrian Palliative Care Society. https://www.ascirs.at

33. Joint Committee on Assisted Dying. Final report of the Joint Committee on Assisted Dying. March 2024. https://data.oireachtas.ie/ie/oireachtas/committee/dail/33/joint_committee_on_assisted_dying/reports/2024/2024-03-20_final-report-of-the-joint-committee-on-assisted-dying_en.pdf

34. Dáil passes vote on assisted dying report. https://www.bbc.co.uk/news/articles/c8rlx84pee2o

35. Montanari Vergallo G, Gulino M. End-of-life care and assisted suicide: an update on the Italian situation from the perspective of the European Court of Human Rights. Ethics Med Public Health. 2022;21:100752.

36. Riva L. The physician-assisted suicide pathway in Italy: ethical assessment and safeguard approaches. J Bioeth Inq. 2024;21(1):185–192.

37. Tuscany becomes Italy's first region to approve assisted suicide for people with incurable illnesses. https://www.euronews.com/health/2025/02/14/tuscany-becomes-italys-first-region-to-approve-assisted-suicide-for-people-with-incurable-

38. Portuguese parliament votes to allow limited euthanasia. https://www.bbc.co.uk/news/world-europe-65574311

39. Cordeiro-Rodrigues L, Wareham CS. Not intrinsically unconstitutional: the Portuguese constitutional court, the right to life, and assisted death. Ethics Global Polit. 2024;17:1–8.

40. Gouveia A. Navigating autonomy and decision-making capacity: legal and ethical considerations in Medical Assistance in Dying for individuals with mental disorders in Portugal. Death Stud. 2025;49(7):850–859.

41. Lewis P. How do permissive regimes regulate assisted dying? In: Board R, Bennett MI, Lewis P, Wagstaff J, Selby P, eds. End-of-life choices for cancer patients. An international perspective. Oxford: EBN Health, 2020.

42. Wels J, Hamarat N. Incidence and prevalence of reported euthanasia cases in Belgium, 2002 to 2023. JAMA Netw Open. 2025;8(4):e256841.

43. Archer M, Willmott L, Chambaere K, et al. Key challenges in providing assisted dying in Belgium: a qualitative analysis of health professionals' experiences. Palliat Care Soc Pract. 2025;19:26323524251318044.

44. Government of the Netherlands. Is euthanasia legal in the Netherlands? https://www.government.nl/topics/euthanasia/is-euthanasia-allowed

45. 2024 report of the Regional Euthanasia Review Committees in the Netherlands. https://www.euthanasiecommissie.nl/documenten/2024/03/24/index

46. Regional Euthanasia Review Committee. Ten percent more reports of euthanasia in 2024. https://www.euthanasiecommissie.nl/actueel/nieuws/2025/03/24/tien-procent-meer-meldingen-euthanasie-in-2024

47. Schweren LJS, Rasing SPA, Kammeraat M, et al. Requests for medical assistance in dying by young Dutch people with psychiatric disorders. JAMA Psychiatry. 2025;82(3):246–252.

48. Campbell S, Denburg A, Moola F, et al. Re-examining medical assistance in dying for mature minors in Canada: reflections for health leaders. Healthc Manage Forum. 2023;36(3):170–175.

49. Campbell S, Cernat A, Denburg A, et al. Exploring assisted dying policies for mature minors: a cross jurisdiction comparison of the Netherlands, Belgium & Canada. Health Policy. 2024;149:105172.

50. Verhofstadt M, Marijnissen R, Creemers D, et al. Exploring the interplay of clinical, ethical and societal dynamics: two decades of Medical Assistance in Dying (MAID) on psychiatric grounds in the Netherlands and Belgium. Front Psychiatry. 2024;15:1463813.

51. Renckens SC, Onwuteaka-Philipsen BD, van der Heide A, et al. Physicians' views on the role of relatives in euthanasia and physician-assisted suicide decision-making: a mixed-methods study among physicians in the Netherlands. BMC Med Ethics. 2024;25(1):43.

52. Asscher E, Metselaar S. Ethical expertise before and after medically assisted dying: the informal and formal role of the ethicist in the Netherlands. Bioethics. 2025;1–8. https://doi.org/10.1111/bioe.13437.

53. Holzman TJ. Creating a safer and better functioning system: Lessons to be learned from the Netherlands for an ethical defence of an autonomy-only approach to assisted dying. Bioethics. 2024;38:558–565.

54. Appel JE, van Wijngaarden E, Dezutter J. Tiredness of life – conceptualizing a complex phenomenon. Psychol Rep. 2024:332941241268815.

55. van der Steen JT, Scheeres-Feitsma TM, Schaafsma P. Commentary to: "Timely dying in dementia: use patients' judgments and broaden the concept of suffering." Timely dying, suffering in dementia, and a role for family and professional caregivers in preventing it. Alzheimers Dement (Amst). 2024;16(1):e12536.

56. Septième rapport à l'attention de la Chambre des Députés (Années 2021 et 2022). https://santesecu.public.lu/dam-assets/fr/publications/r/rapport-loi-euthanasie-2021-2022/rapport-loi-euthanasie-2021-2022.pdf

57. Kozlov E, Nowels M, Gusmano M, et al. Aggregating 23 years of data on medical aid in dying in the United States. J Am Geriatr Soc. 2022;70(10):3040–3044.

58. Grubbs KH, Keinath CM, Biggar SE. A rapid review of medical assistance in dying in the United States and its Implications for practice for health care professionals. Rapid Rev. 2024;26:296–302.

59. Pottash M, Saikaly K, Stevenson M, et al. A survey of clinicians who provide aid in dying.. Am J Hosp Palliat Care. 2024;41(9):1045–1050.

60. Harrawood KA. Medical aid in dying: the role of the nurse practitioner. J Am Assoc Nurse Pract. 2024;36(8):426–430.

61. Regnard C, Worthington A, Finlay I. Oregon death with dignity act access: 25-year analysis. BMJ Support Palliat Care. 2024;14(4):455–461.

62. Kious BM. Medical assistance in dying in neurology. Neurol Clin. 2023;41:443–454.

63. Macmillan P, Hughes S, Loscar A, et al. The pharmacology of aid in dying: from database analyses to evidence-based best practices. J Palliat Med. 2025;28(4):492–498.

64. CAPC About the Center to Advance Palliative Care. Available from: https://www.capc.org/about/capc/ (accessed 15 August 2025).

65. CAPC America's readiness to meet the needs of people with serious illness a state-by-state look at palliative care capacity. 2024 serious illness scorecard. Available from: https://scorecard.capc.org/wp-content/uploads/2024/11/CAPC-Serious-Illness-Scorecard-Report.pdf (accessed 15 August 2025).

Chapter 5: International Assisted Dying Laws and Practice: Canada

In Canada, AD is usually referred to as Medical Assistance in Dying, MAiD. In Canada, currently MAiD is based on the relief of intolerable suffering and does not carry a requirement for a diagnosis of a terminal illness with a predicted period of life expectancy in all cases. To understand the current healthcare status and eligibility for AD/MAiD in Canada, it is necessary to describe the legislative processes which have shaped the current status. In February 2015, the Canadian Supreme Court judged the case of *Carter v. Canada* and found that the previous criminal code ruling that it was a crime to assist someone to die, violated the *Charter of Rights and Freedoms*. The Supreme Court's view was that people with grievous and irremediable medical conditions had a right to access AD. It gave the Canadian Parliament time to introduce legislation. In 2016, the Canadian Federal Parliament passed a Bill to legalise AD. The 2016 Bill specified "enduring and intolerable suffering" and that the diagnosis meant that death was reasonably foreseeable-- thus using the "terminal illness" framework for eligibility.[1,2]

The restriction of the Canadian Law to the "terminal illness" framework was challenged legally in British Columbia and in Quebec. It was argued that the restriction to a reasonably foreseeable time of death excluded people with long term medical conditions who were suffering intolerably but whose life expectancy could not be estimated. The Supreme Courts of British Columbia and Quebec upheld these arguments in a judgement known as "Truchon" and the Federal Government accepted that further legal changes were required.[3]

Updated law in 2020/2021

In 2020, Canada introduced an *Act to amend the Criminal Code (medical assistance in dying)*. This was shaped by the Truchon case where the "reasonable foreseeability of natural death" eligibility criterion was found to be unconstitutional. The changes were also informed by Canada's experience with MAiD and feedback from over 300,000 people and 120 experts in consultations. In 2021, changes to the legislation took effect that:

- Revised eligibility criteria for obtaining MAiD and the process of assessment.
- Changed existing safeguards for eligible people whose natural death is considered reasonably foreseeable.
- Expanded the framework for federal data collection and reporting.

The revised law contains new safeguards for eligible people who request medical assistance in dying and whose death is **not** considered reasonably foreseeable.

Eligibility for MaiD for patients with solely mental illness

The inclusion of mental illness including dementia as eligible in the Canadian MAiD legislation has proved challenging for all concerned. The inclusion of mental illness as eligible for MAiD was permitted initially if it was regarded as grievous and irremediable. This was due to take effect in

2023. However, it was concluded that more time is required, and the issue has been put back to 2027. The future for this change in the Federal law appears uncertain and the approach in Quebec is currently also uncertain. The Quebec Provincial government plans to include mental illness eligibility and advanced directives for people who have early dementia.[4–6]

The current status of MAiD in Canada

The implementation of MAiD in Canada since 2020 is summarised for patients by the Canadian Government website.[7] The two methods of medical assistance in dying available in Canada remain that a physician or nurse practitioner directly administers a substance that causes death, such as an injection of a drug, or a physician or nurse practitioner provides or prescribes a drug that the eligible person takes themselves, to bring about their own death.

Healthcare professionals are permitted to suggest MAiD to a patient.

To be eligible for medical assistance in dying, patients must meet all the following criteria.

- Be eligible for health services funded by a province or territory, or the federal government.
- Be at least 18 years old and mentally competent.
- Have a grievous and irremediable medical condition.
- Make a voluntary request for medical assistance in dying which cannot be the result of outside pressure or influence.
- Give informed consent to receive medical assistance in dying.

To be considered as having a grievous and irremediable medical condition, a patient must meet all of the following criteria:

- Have a serious illness, disease, or disability.
- Be in an advanced state of decline that cannot be reversed.
- Experience unbearable physical or mental suffering from the illness, disease, disability or state of decline that cannot be relieved under conditions that are considered acceptable.

In Canada, a patient does not need to have a fatal or terminal condition to be eligible for medical assistance in dying. Patients with only a mental illness are not eligible for medical assistance in dying.

The process of consent, providing information, and confirming eligibility are closely defined and may vary between Provinces. Procedural safeguards include two independent medical assessments confirming the patient has an incurable grievous and irremediable medical condition that is in an advanced state of irreversible decline, and that the patient is capable of receiving and willing to receive euthanasia. A written request must be signed by an independent witness who must confirm that there has been no coercion. Withdrawal of consent at any time in any manner is allowed and a final consent before receiving medical assistance in dying is required. Witnesses and healthcare workers must have no financial or legal interest in the case. Consent must be expressed and not implied. Request and withdrawal of request can be repeated. They must also meet extra safeguards if death is not naturally foreseeable. It is possible to waive the requirement to provide consent just before the receipt of medical assistance in dying, only if natural death is reasonably foreseeable and while the person has decision-making capacity.

It is possible to make a written arrangement with a practitioner so that they can administer medical assistance in dying in the event of failed self-administration. This arrangement allows for clinician-administered medical assistance in dying if there are complications during self-administration that cause loss of decision-making capacity but not death. A medical practitioner must be present at the time of the self-administration of the medications.

If the medical practitioners assessing a request for MAiD determine that death is not reasonably foreseeable, there are extra safeguards that must be met before medical assistance in dying can be provided:

1. One of the two medical practitioners who provides an assessment must have expertise in the medical condition that is causing unbearable suffering.

2. Patients must be informed of available means to relieve suffering and offered consultations with professionals who provide such services.

3. Patients and practitioners must have discussed reasonable and available means to relieve suffering, and all agree that the person has seriously considered those means.

4. The eligibility assessment must take a minimum of 90 days, unless the assessments have been completed sooner and there is an immediate risk of losing capacity to consent.

5. Immediately before medical assistance in dying, the practitioner must:
   - Give an opportunity to withdraw request.
   - Ensure that express consent to receive medical assistance in dying is given.

Canada's law does not permit minors access AD.

In 2020, Rodin et al.[8] summarised the first three years of Canadian experience with MAiD. "*MAiD has become a prevalent practice in Canada, with varying degrees of integration into mainstream medical systems in the first 3 years since its inception. During this period, more than 7000 people in Canada chose to end their lives through AD, representing approximately 1% of deaths in this country and almost 2% of cancer-related deaths. In some respects, Canadian MAiD statistics mirror those in other jurisdictions, with almost two-thirds of requests for MAiD coming from individuals with cancer. There have been lessons learned and unresolved issues identified related to MAiD in Canada. The latter include how soon before the end-of-life MAiD should be delivered, whether it should be made available to mature minors and to the psychiatrically ill and whether it should be delivered based on an advance directive of patients who are no longer competent at the time of its delivery*".

The fifth annual report on Medical Assistance in Dying

In 2023, the fifth annual report on Medical Assistance in Dying (MAiD,[9]) in Canada provides a summary of MAiD requests, assessments and provisions for the 2023 calendar year.[9] While the number of MAiD provisions increased in 2023, the rate of growth was halved over previous years.

There were 60,301 MAiD deaths 2016–2023 with 15,343 in 2023, 4.7% of all deaths in Canada; average age was 77.6 years. In 2022, the underlying medical conditions included cancer (63%), cardiovascular (18.8%), and neurological conditions (12.6%). The trend 2016–2023 was

2016	1018
2017	2838
2018	4493
2019	5665

2020	7611
2021	10,092
2022	13,241
2023	15,343

There were 19,660 MAiD requests in 2023. 15,343 received MAiD; 2906 died before receiving MAiD; 915 individuals were deemed ineligible, and 496 individuals withdrew their request. The number of MAiD provisions in 2023 represents an increase of 15.8% over 2022. This represents a slowing over previous years (2019–2022) which had an average growth rate of approximately 31%.

This report provides insights into the circumstances of people receiving MAiD under two separate "tracks":

- Those in "Track 1" who met the eligibility criteria set out above and were assessed as having a natural death that was "reasonably foreseeable."
- Those in "Track 2" who met the eligibility criteria set out above and were assessed as having a natural death that was not "reasonably foreseeable."

Most MAiD provisions (95.9%; $n = 14,721$) were for individuals in Track 1; 4.1% ($n = 622$) of MAiD provisions were for individuals in Track 2. Those who received MAiD under Track 1 were older, and more likely to have cancer as an underlying medical condition. Those receiving MAiD under Track 2 were predominantly women, slightly younger, and lived with their illness for a much longer period. People who receive MAiD do not disproportionately come from lower-income or disadvantaged communities. Most MAiD recipients who required either palliative care or disability support services received these services or had access to them.

MAiD appears to be becoming an area of focussed expertise for some practitioners.

- There were 2200 unique MAiD practitioners in 2023. The majority (94.5%) were physicians, while 5.5% were nurse practitioners.
- A group of 89 practitioners were responsible for 35.1% of all Track 1 and 28.6% of all Track 2 cases, respectively.

Close et al.[10] looked at 15 available practice standards and related documents across Canada reporting that most described the legislation without guidance on how it should be applied. Regulators do provide guidance in areas of medical practice such as competencies, required documentation and patient centred care. Rights of conscientious objectors were covered. The regulatory practice standards and guidance documents for MAiD can vary across Canada in different Provinces.[10] Guidance may outline the law without giving clarity on how it may be applied.[10]

In 2023, following the work of an Expert Panel, the MAiD Practice Standards Task Group was set up[11] in order *"That the Government of Canada, in partnership with provinces and territories, continue to facilitate the collaboration of regulatory authorities, medical practitioners and nurse practitioners to establish standards for medical practitioners and nurse practitioners for the purpose of assessing MAiD requests, with a view to harmonising access to MAiD across Canada".* The Task Group has produced two key advisory documents

- Model Practice Standard for Medical Assistance in Dying[12]
- Advice to the Profession: Medical Assistance in Dying[13]

which are intended to provide a consistent framework of advice to be taken up by the responsible authorities in the Canadian Provinces. Education and training developments are a key part of developing high quality consistent AD services and a skilled workforce and these are addressed in Canada through the Canadian MAiD Curriculum.[14,15]

Health cost implications

The Canadian Federal Government carried out an estimation of the cost implications of the introduction of the first phase of AD up to 2020 when the eligibility criteria included "foreseeable life expectancy" and then also the implications of the 2020/2021 changes which broadened the eligibility criteria.[16] The costs of healthcare in Canada are covered by the Provincial Governments. In the first phase they estimated that the gross reduction in health care costs would amount to $109.2 million with MAiD costing an estimated at $22.3 million, a net cost reduction of $86.9 million. For the changes introduced in 2020/2021 they estimated a further net reduction of health care costs for provincial governments of an estimated 0.08% of provincial health care budgets. These figures are at best rough estimates and do not constitute a formal health economic evaluation. However, they have been used to infer both that cost reduction is an unacceptable motivation behind AD or that the case for AD is strengthened if there is no expectation of any extra healthcare cost. They do suggest that any healthcare cost implication is likely to be marginal and that cost-based arguments should not take a central role in considering legislation to permit or modify AD in new jurisdictions.

Current Canadian public opinion

A 2023 survey by the Angus Reid Institute showed 61% of Canadians supported the current legislation, while 31% supported extending AD to mental disorders.[16] Choi et al.[17] showed that it is, however, important to have clear, sometimes detailed, questions to ensure that the opinions provided give a genuine reflection of the respondents understanding of the issues around a highly complex subject like MAiD.[18]

Disability and disadvantage

The international literature on Disability and Disadvantage is discussed in Chapter 8. Canadian commentators have expressed the views that the MAiD provisions and implementation may disadvantage impoverished and disabled people[19-21] although the 2023 data do not show that there is an overrepresentation of MAiD recipients from poor backgrounds or that disabled people are overrepresented among MAiD recipients. Commentators report that the Disability community feels ignored in the discussions of MAiD and its proposed expansions and some legal challenges have been entered.[22,23] Berube et al.[24] surveyed 966 responders in Quebec to assess their knowledge and attitudes about end-of-life care and MAiD. People facing social and economic challenges knew less about end-of-life practices but had a positive attitude to MAiD. Lund[25] comments that the Disability community has been historically divided on MAiD with some seeing it as an example of able people undervaluing the lives of disabled people ("ableism") and others viewing it as it provided an option for self-determination.[25] Asada et al. gives a comprehensive overview of where there are potential risks that disabled or disadvantaged people could suffer from a lack of access to MAiD when they are eligible and may wish to make that choice, or that they may be at risk of pressure to take up such a choice inappropriately. The importance of careful and detailed prospective investigation of the interaction between disadvantage, disability and MAiD is necessary and justified.[26]

Patient and family experience

These aspects of AD are reviewed in Chapter 9. Canadian studies included:

- The grief experienced by families after a loved one is lost through MAiD is similar in its nature and severity to that following a natural death with palliative care.[27]
- Discordance between family members about a decision to access MAiD complicate the process of MAiD and bereavement.[28]
- Caregivers and patients can be a valuable source of suggestion for improving the regulation of AD.[29]
- While families frequently express gratitude for the availability of MAiD, the day on which MAiD occurs can be "jarring and unsettling" and an active approach to involving family members, with careful preparation and a degree of ceremony can have a positive impact of their experience.[30]

Healthcare professional experience

These aspects of AD are reviewed in Chapter 7. Canadian studies included:

- Bustin et al.[31] systematically reviewed the role of nurses in AD in Canada, New Zealand and Australia highlighting the complexity of the decision making and the moral, philosophical and social influences involved, calling for developments in education and training for these roles.
- Wibisono et al.,[32] with collaborators in Australia, the US and UK systematically reviewed the evidence on the impact of involvement in AD upon the mental health of healthcare professionals. They found no evidence for an association between participation in AD services and anxiety or moral distress. Winters et al.[33] studied the impact of MAiD participation specifically upon Canadian healthcare professionals in the first 2 years after its introduction and found positive reactions to providing autonomy to patients and relieving their suffering while they were also experiencing tensions around their professional duties and balancing their own needs.
- Winters et al.[34] also reported the way that Canadian healthcare professionals, specifically physicians, described their roles in in the MAiD process. This covered a range from the "conduit" role in which they gave the main, moral decisions to the patient and focussed on guiding them through the complex process of MAiD to the "conductor" role where they felt they shared to decisions more closely and supported the patient's decision-making process through their professional judgement.
- Canadian investigators and physicians were involved in the international studies of physicians own views and preferences for end-of-life care reported by Mroz et al.[35,36] In 1157, survey responses from across the world, about half of the physicians consider AD as a good or very good option ranging from 40% in Italy to 81% in Belgium for a cancer scenario. They reported that their own preferences do influence the advice they offer to patients.

Rodin, Shapiro, Wales and Li[8] concluded *"The experience of AD in Canada indicates that an intervention such as MAiD, which generated polarised and heated debate, can be implemented and normalised within a relatively short period of time. MAiD continues to be facilitated and provided by physicians and nurse practitioners from diverse specialties, and robust professional organisations have emerged to support those involved in this activity. MAiD has not been formally supported by palliative care organisations and bodies in Canada, but the assessment and delivery of MAiD now occurs alongside palliative care and the process frequently involves palliative care physicians, nurses and settings. Further, the legalisation and introduction of MAiD may be seen to reflect the democratisation of decision making in end-of-life care, which may be the most remarkable aspect of AD in Canada and elsewhere."*

The experience of Canada is highly relevant to jurisdictions which are introducing the option for AD at the present time. The interplay of legal, political and healthcare issues is complex and requires constant review. The evolution of the eligibility for MAiD has been rapid and there have been several challenging legal, political and healthcare episodes. Constant vigilance, monitoring and reporting are essential to ensure a safe and effective service.

The debate around MAiD and mental illness remains active. The inclusion of intolerable suffering due to mental health diagnoses as a sole eligibility criterion for MAiD is controversial in Canada.[37,38] The definition of what constitutes "irremediability" and the links between mental health disorders and the patient's relationships, socioeconomic circumstances and their access to high quality healthcare remains to be resolved. The political difficulties in developing provisions for mental health including dementia are clearly shown by delays and the disagreement between Quebec and the Federal Canadian Government.[39]

Rodin et al commented *"The experience in Canada has highlighted the importance of a systemic and systematic approach to educating patients and all healthcare providers in the introduction of MAiD and the need for national oversight and review of the practice.[8]"*

Are there lessons in the Canadian experience for jurisdictions which are contemplating legalising AD? The Canadian system moved from a "terminal illness" based set of criteria to a set of criteria which includes "intolerable suffering without a foreseeable life expectancy" within 5 years driven by court rulings. This is not comparable to proposed UK legislation where any such changes would require primary legislation with the appropriate public, professional and parliamentary debate. However, despite this fundamental difference, there are lessons to be learned from Canadian experience. Notes of caution come from

- The speed of increase in the proportion of people accessing AD. This has grown more rapidly than the international averages and reached levels seen only in the Benelux countries in Europe, reflecting the eligibility criteria in Canada and the AD options available.

- The speed with which the eligibility criteria were altered as a result of court rulings on legal rights. The fact that delays were necessary to intended legislation in the eligibility of people with suffering solely from mental health disorders, illustrates this issue.

- Different jurisdictions in Canada, notable the Federal Government and the Quebec Provincial Government, formed different views on the required legislation, which is unlikely to provide a concerned observer with confidence.

- Operational details and guidance have been different in different Provinces suggesting such guidance should be available before an implementation plan is made. A National training curriculum is also an early requirement of a successful system.

- Workload and work stresses are a common theme in reports of the experiences of healthcare professionals

On a more positive side the data suggest that the Canadian healthcare systems have been

- The Canadian systems have been able to cope with an increase in the proportion of AD among total deaths which is higher than the international averages in permissive jurisdictions

- Reported patient/ family/ informal caregiver experiences have commonly been positive and the Canadian public remain supportive of AD after the experience to date.

- There is no evidence so far of an inappropriate uptake of AD among disadvantaged people, although continued meticulous monitoring is clearly required to maintain their confidence
- Over time there has been engagement with the procedures involved in AD from a wide range of healthcare disciplines and a degree of specialisation in the delivery of services is discernible.

References

1. An Act to amend the Criminal Code and to make related amendments to other Acts (medical assistance in dying). https://openparliament.ca/bills/42-1/C-14/

2. Doctor-assisted dying bill restricted to adults facing 'foreseeable' death. https://www.cbc.ca/news/politics/canada-physician-assisted-death-law-1.3535193

3. Legislative Background: Bill C-7: Government of Canada's Legislative Response to the Superior Court of Québec *Truchon* Decision. https://www.justice.gc.ca/eng/csj-sjc/pl/ad-am/c7/p1.html

4. Final Report of the Expert Panel on MAiD and Mental Illness. https://www.canada.ca/en/health-canada/corporate/about-health-canada/public-engagement/external-advisory-bodies/expert-panel-maid-mental-illness/final-report-expert-panel-maid-mental-illness.html

5. Delay of eligibility for medical assistance in dying for persons suffering solely from mental illness proposed by Ministers of Justice and Health. https://www.canada.ca/en/department-justice/news/2023/02/delay-of-eligibility-for-medical-assistance-in-dying-for-persons-suffering-solely-from-mental-illness-proposed-by-ministers-of-justice-and-health.html

6. Dyer O. Canada shelves plan to allow medically assisted dying for people with mental illness. BMJ 2024;384q:271.

7. Medical Assistance in dying. Government of Canada. Last Modified in 2024. https://www.canada.ca/en/health-canada/services/health-services-benefits/medical-assistance-dying.html

8. Rodin G, Shapiro G, Wales J, et al. Assisted dying in Canada: lessons from the first 3 years. In: Board R, Bennett MI, Lewis P, Wagstaff J, Selby P, eds. End of life choices for cancer patients. An international perspective. Oxford: EBN Health, 2020.

9. The Fifth Annual Report on Medical Assistance in Dying (MAID) in Canada https://www.canada.ca/en/health-canada/services/publications/health-system-services/annual-report-medical-assistance-dying-2023.html

10. Close E, Gupta M, Downie J, et al. Medical assistance in dying in Canada: a review of regulatory practice standards and guidance documents for physicians. Palliat Care Soc Pract. 2025;19:26323524251338859.

11. Background Document: The Work of the Medical Assistance in Dying (MAID) Practice Standards Task Group. https://www.canada.ca/en/health-canada/services/publications/health-system-services/background-document-work-medical-assistance-dying-practice-standards-task-group.html

12. MAID Practice Standard Task Group. Model Practice Standard for Medical Assistance in Dying (MAID). Canada: Health Canada. 2023. https://www.canada.ca/en/health-canada/services/publications/health-system-services/model-practice-standard-medical-assistance-dying.html

13. MAID Practice Standards Tasks Group. Advice to the Profession: Medical Assistance in Dying (MAID). Canada: Health Canada. 2023. https://www.canada.ca/content/dam/hc-sc/documents/services/medical-assistance-dying/advice-profession/advice-profession.pdf

14. Shapiro GK, Hunt K, Braund H, et al. Development of a Canadian medical assistance in dying curriculum for healthcare providers. J Med Educ Curric Dev. 2024;11:23821205241272376.

15. Canadian MAiD curriculum. https://camapcanada.ca/curriculum

16. Cost estimate for Bill C-7 "Medical Assistance In Dying". 2020. https://qsarchive-archiveqs. pbo-dpb.ca/web/default/files/Documents/Reports/RP-2021-025-M/RP-2021-025-M_en.pdf

17. Canadians supportive of assisted dying law but wary of mental health expansion: poll. https://globalnews.ca/news/9479497/canada-assisted-dying-mental-health-poll/

18. Choi WJW, Astrachan IM, Sinaii N, et al. When medical assistance in dying is not a last resort option: survey of the Canadian public. BMJ Open. 2024;14(6):e087736.

19. Why is Canada euthanising the poor? https://www.spectator.co.uk/article/most-read-2022-why-is-canada-euthanising-the-poor

20. How poverty, not pain, is driving Canadians with disabilities to consider medically assisted death. https://globalnews.ca/news/9176485/poverty-canadians-disabilities-medically-assisted-death

21. Grant I. Legislated ableism: Bill C-7 and the rapid expansion of MAiD in Canada, 2023. https://papers.ssrn.com/sol3/papers.cfm?abstract_id=4544454

22. Chown S. Disability community feels ignored in Canada's assisted dying expansion. BMJ. 2024;385:q806.

23. Dyer O. Assisted dying: disability advocates launch legal challenge to Canada's law. BMJ. 2024;387:q2161.

24. Bérubé A, Tapp D, Dupéré S, et al. Do socioeconomic factors influence knowledge, attitudes, and representations of end-of-life practices? A cross-sectional study. J Palliat Care. 2025;40(2):152–161.

25. Lund EM. Advocacy considerations regarding medical aid in dying for people with nonterminal chronic illnesses and disabilities. Rehabil Psychol. 2025;70(2):119–122.

26. Asada Y, Campbell LA, Grignon M, et al. mportance of investigating vulnerabilities in health and social service provision among requestors of medical assistance in dying. Lancet Reg Health Am. 2024;35:100810.

27. Laperle P, Achille M, Ummel D. To lose a loved one by medical assistance in dying or by natural death with palliative care: a mixed methods comparison of grief experiences. Omega (Westport). 2024;89(3):931–953.

28. Serota K, Buchman DZ, Atkinson M. Mapping MAiD discordance: a qualitative analysis of the factors complicating MAiD bereavement in Canada. Qual Health Res. 2024;34(3):195–204.

29. Jeanneret R, Close E, Willmott L, et al. Patients' and caregivers' suggestions for improving assisted dying regulation: a qualitative study in Australia and Canada. Health Expect. 2024;27(3):e14107.

30. Nissim R, Chu P, Stere A, et al. "Walk me through the final day": a thematic analysis study on the family caregiver experience of the Medical Assistance in Dying procedure day. Palliat Med. 2024;38(6):660–668.

31. Bustin H, Jamieson I, Seay C, et al. A meta-synthesis exploring nurses' experiences of assisted dying and participation decision-making. J Clin Nurs. 2024;33(2):710–723.

32. Wibisono S, Minto K, Lizzio-Wilson M, et al. Attitudes toward and experience with assisted-death services and psychological implications for health practitioners: a narrative systematic review. Omega (Westport). 2025;91(2):590–612.

33. Winters JP, Jaye C, Pickering NJ, e al. Providing medically assisted dying in Canada: a qualitative study of emotional and moral impact. J Med Ethics. 2025;51(6):400–410.

34. Winters JP, Walker S, Pickering NJ, et al. Conduit or conductor? Physician providers' descriptions of their role as MAiD assessors in the first years after legalisation in Canada. J Med Ethics. 2025:jme-2024-110518.

35. Mroz S, Dierickx S, Chambaere K, et al. Physicians' preferences for their own end of life: a comparison across North America, Europe, and Australia. J Med Ethics. 2025:jme-2024-110192.

36. Mroz S, Daenen F, Dierickx S, et al. Associations between physicians' personal preferences for end-of-life decisions and their own clinical practice: PROPEL survey study in Europe, North America, and Australia. Palliat Med. 2025;39(2):266–276.

37. Bojkovic K, Jupudi R, Bojkovic M, et al. The right to life, and death: a health equity approach to canada's expansion of medical assistance in dying for individuals with mental disorder(s). Omega (Westport). 2025:302228251318414.

38. Hawke LD, Bastidas-Bilbao H, Cappe V, et al. MAiD study team at the centre for addiction and mental health. medical assistance in dying for mental illness as a sole underlying medical condition and its relationship to suicide: a qualitative lived experience-engaged study [Aide Médicale à Mourir Pour Maladie Mentale Comme Seule Condition Médicale Sous-Jacente et Son Lien Avec le Suicide: Une Etude Qualitative Engagée Dans l'Expérience Vécue]. Can J Psychiatry. 2024;69(5):314–325.

39. Dyer O. Assisted dying: Quebec allows advance directives, defying federal ban. BMJ. 2024;386:q2029.

Chapter 6: International Assisted Dying Laws and Practice: New Zealand and Australia

New Zealand and the individual States of Australia introduced legislation to permit AD at the end of the last decade and have now some 5 years' experience of its implementation and delivery. The eligibility criteria for AD in the Australasian countries are very similar to those proposed for the UK and British Isles.

New Zealand

Assisted Dying has been permitted in New Zealand since November 2021 under the End-of-Life Choice Act 2019 and a binding referendum.[1] It is available to New Zealanders with unbearable suffering from a terminal illness that is likely to end their life within 6 months. It has a formal assessment with strict criteria and safeguards. A person with a terminal illness may request medication to end their life. The process and eligibility are set out on the Health New Zealand website[2] which says

*"There are strict eligibility criteria for assisted dying. Not everyone with a terminal illness will be eligible for assisted dying. The Act states that to be eligible, the person must **meet all of the criteria.** The person must be:*

- *aged 18 years or over*
- *a citizen or permanent resident of New Zealand*
- *suffering from a terminal illness that is likely to end their life within 6 months*
- *in an advanced state of irreversible decline in physical capability*
- *experiencing unbearable suffering that cannot be relieved in a manner that the person considers tolerable*
- *competent to make an informed decision about assisted dying.*

A person cannot access assisted dying solely because they have a mental disorder or mental illness, have a disability or are of advanced age. However, people with these conditions may be eligible to access assisted dying if they meet the eligibility criteria.

Whether or not a particular person's illness or condition meets the eligibility criteria is determined on a case-by-case basis, considering all of the person's individual clinical circumstances including the severity and prognosis of the illness(es) they are experiencing.

Having a particular illness does not automatically make a person eligible for assisted dying. Similarly, having a particular diagnosis, illness or disability does not automatically rule out assisted dying as an option. Every person's clinical situation is different. Medical practitioners involved in the service will assess if a person meets the eligibility criteria during the application process in the first instance."

The decision to have an assisted death must be made by the person with a terminal illness. A health practitioner is not permitted to raise this option with a patient unprompted. The medication may be taken orally or given intravenously by a healthcare professional depending on the patient's preference.

The Support and Consultation for End of Life in New Zealand Group (SCENZ) Group[3] is a statutory group established under the End-of-Life Choice Act 2019 which maintains a list of health practitioners willing to provide AD services and is responsible for clinical guidelines and the standard of care for AD in New Zealand.

Three annual reports have documented the implementation of the change in the law.[4–6] The first 2 years of the operation of the new law saw a quite rapid increase in the numbers of applications in 2021/2022 to about 60 per month. This remained roughly constant in 2023. Data for the period April 2023 to March 2024 suggest an increase of 11%. Over that period, there were 834 new formal applications for AD and 334 people had an assisted death in that period.

In 2024, the NZ Ministry of Health conducted a review of the End-of-Life Choice Act[7] and its principal conclusions were

> **"The End-of-Life Choice Act is achieving its primary purpose**
>
> *The End-of-Life Choice Act 2019 (the Act) has largely been operating well and has achieved its primary purpose of giving people with a terminal illness who meet certain criteria the option to request and receive medical assistance to end their lives. More than 2400 people have requested an assisted death, and more than 970 have received an assisted death since the Act came into force on 7 November 2021.*
>
> *The core processes in the Act to apply, be assessed for, and receive an assisted death are clear and robust. The eligibility requirements to receive an assisted death are also reasonably clear, noting that some of these criteria involve a level of subjectivity in the judgements that practitioners must make when they are assessing people.*
>
> *The intended limitations on people seeking an assisted death are also clear in the wording of the legislation – that the decision to seek an assisted death must be made by the individual, that a person cannot receive an assisted death if they do not meet the eligibility criteria, and an assisted death cannot be approved or consented to in advance.*
>
> *The additional scrutiny provided by the Registrar has been a valuable safeguard in the process.*
>
> *The practical provision of assisted dying has also worked well. There is an effective and responsive workforce that is well supported by the Assisted Dying Service. Funding of the service has supported access to assisted dying and supported practitioners to travel to people who are often not able to travel themselves.*
>
> *The level of compliance with requirements in the Act has also been very high, though there have been a small number of potential breaches. The Ministry is confident that everyone who has received an assisted death met the eligibility requirements set out in the Act and had chosen an assisted death.*
>
> **There is scope for improvement to the Act across a number of areas**
>
> *The End-of-Life Choice Act is a relatively new piece of legislation, seeking to regulate a complex and sensitive health service that is new to New Zealand society and the health system.*
>
> *While the Act has enabled people to access assisted dying, there are a number of areas where the Ministry considers that changes could be made to improve the operation of the Act. These are organised into five areas:*
>
> - *Supporting access and safety.*
> - *Improving the process to receive assisted dying.*
> - *Aligning the Act with the wider health system.*

- *Ensuring a capable and effective workforce for assisted dying.*
- *Clarifying organisational roles and responsibilities in the Act.*

In each of these areas, the Ministry has identified a number of issues that have come up during the review process.

Recommendations are made in each area that the Ministry considers would address the issues discussed and improve the operation and effectiveness of the Act in achieving its purposes. Many of these recommendations are interconnected and mutually supporting".

The New Zealand Review[7] provides a model for the detailed level of monitoring and improvement of AD processes and implementation. Issues identified by the review were:

1. Supporting access and safety

Not allowing healthcare professionals to raise assisted dying created a significant barrier and limited information being available. The term used to require practitioners to "do their best" to detect if patients were under pressure to access AD was poorly defined. Assessing mental competence may be needed at more than one point in time. The expected duties of the HCPs were insufficiently defined. The approach to defining breaches which could be criminal or could be less serious was set out clearly. Specific guidance on what might be published about assisted deaths was needed.

2. Improving the process

The procedures for declining AD and making a second request were unclear. The procedures for handovers to another HCP when one could not continue were not clear. The time period during which a person could receive AD once they were deemed eligible was not sufficiently clear and rules for setting and moving dates were found unhelpful. The level of operational detail set out in the Act was felt to be high and possibly unhelpful.

3. Aligning with the wider health system

There were challenges aligning the AD service with the wider healthcare system. The Act allows conscientious objection for HCPs but there may be a need to more clearly set out that such objections should not lead to obstruction or active dissuasion. The role of care facilities is not defined. Some institutions have created barriers to access to AD.

4. Workforce

The threshold at which HCPs can provide AD may have been set too low and there is no legal requirement to complete training. The workforce has been too small. Nurse practitioners' roles are vital but are limited to the final stages of the procedure making continuity in care difficult. HCPs involved in AD need ongoing support.

5. Organisational roles

Issues were identified with the definitions of the roles of SCENZ, the role of the Registrar in checking compliance and the scope of the Review Committee.

The Review Committee made 25 recommendations and 11 minor recommendations for improvements based on the issues reported above and NZ experience covering all aspects of the Act and its implementation.[7]

Dehkhoda et al. in 2025 reported 22 interviews with healthcare professional workers (HCPs) who had been involved in the implementation of AD in New Zealand.[8] Most were General

Practitioners, and their experience ranged from 3 to 30 AD cases. The researchers identified a theoretical framework around "knowing, experience and practice" which they developed to explore the interviewees experiences and collected them under "Knowing, Doing and Being". This qualitative study adds insights to the formal information from the high-level Review Committee revealing altruism, the need for training[9] and support, a sense that the legislation had set out a substantial bureaucracy which was quite difficult to cover quickly with very unwell patients. They were challenged by the need for an estimate of life expectancy, confident in their ability to identify mental competence and some were unsure how to measure "unbearable suffering". They reported experience of the option for HCPs to conscientiously object generating barriers for patients. The limitation of HCPs initiating discussions of AD were felt to create barriers for patients. Although the details of the provision of materials to provide AD were felt to need refinement, most HCPs felt that patients and their families appreciated the AD process and the sense of reclaiming control that it provided. It was commonly reported that most patients were white and well educated with a relatively low proportion of Māori patients. Professional stresses and the personal impact of being an HCP who delivers AD were commonly mentioned, with references to s fear of social isolation.

Snelling[10] reported interviews with twenty-six HCPs and a thematic analysis identifying four themes (i) difference in organisational response to AD; (ii) challenges in applying the law; (iii) experiences at the coal face and (iv) functionality of the AD system. This group involved mainly nurses and doctors and included those who had conscientious objections to AD, those who were active supporters and involved in AD and those who had not been in favour of AD but who felt that it had been made legal and was now part of the health care system. A range of organisational responses were described from "proactive and informed" to "heads in sand". Hospices were rarely involved in AD. Most HCPs with conscientious objections were referring patient appropriately. The limitation of HCPs initiating discussions on AD, the clarification of the meaning of "unbearable suffering" and the difficulty of setting and changing dates for AD were again prominent in the interviews.

Most patients preferred the IV route and venous access is a recurring concern. Workforce capacity, the timely working of the system, resources and funding, and the need for training were again prominent.

"The most difficult task" in some cases could be telling a patient who had sought AD that they were ineligible. The authors recognised the early nature of the experience and the expectation that there would be evolution towards improvements and a more settled and routine expectation for AD, as found in other jurisdictions.[11–14]

Bustin et al.[15] systematically reviewed the role of nurses in AD in New Zealand and Australia highlighting the complexity of the decision making and the moral, philosophical and social influences involved, calling for developments in education and training for these roles. Mooney et al.[16] systematically reviewed the literature on assessing patients' decision-making capacity in New Zealand and Australia. In 33 articles, they identified a lack of standardisation and guidelines, the need for more training and the complexities of the professional roles and the medico-legal interface.

Australia

Most Australian legislation and medical literature refer to AD as Voluntary Assisted Dying (VAD). The development of AD legislation in Australia has been complex with most primary legislation being introduced by individual Australian states. For Australian Territories, where federal law can influence legislation for VAD, there has been a complex interaction between Territorial and Federal legislators. However, the situation is now becoming clear.[17] Voluntary Assisted Dying has been legal in Victoria since 2019,[18] Western Australia since 2021,[19] Tasmania 2022,[20] Queensland 2023,[21] South Australia 2023,[22] and New South Wales since 2023.[23] The Australian Capital Territory will initiate an AD scheme in 2025.[24] The Northern Territory is likely to initiate a scheme in the foreseeable future.[25]

Victoria. Victoria was the first state to permit AD in Australia. The bill was modelled on advice from an expert panel and after debate and amendment was passed in 2017 and came into effect in 2019.[26,27] Notably the implementation was on-going over 18 months as processes to ensure eligibility and access were developed and translated into appropriate clinical practice. The legislation VAD in Victoria has generally been a model for that in the rest of Australia. Residents of Victoria who are at least 18 years old with intact decision-making capacity are eligible to apply for AD. Eligibility requires that a person has an incurable, advanced and progressive disease, illness or medical condition with intolerable suffering. Two medical practitioners must indicate that they expect the condition to cause death within 6 months. There is an exception for a person suffering from a neurodegenerative condition where instead the expectation of death must be within 12 months. The medication is prescribed for self-administration unless the patient is unable to take the drugs orally in which case they may be given intravenously by an HCP.

In Victoria, therefore, people can ask for voluntary assisted dying if they meet all the following conditions:

1. They must have an advanced disease that will cause their death and that is:
   - likely to cause their death within 6 months (or within 12 months for neurodegenerative diseases like motor neurone disease)
   - causing the person suffering that is unacceptable to them
2. They must have the ability to make and communicate a decision about voluntary assisted dying throughout the formal request process.
3. They must also:
   - be an adult 18 years or over
   - have been living in Victoria for at least 12 months
   - be an Australian citizen or permanent resident (69)

The oversight of VAD in Victoria sits with the Voluntary Assisted Dying Review Board which most recently reported on July 2024 to June 2024.[27] In the Forward to the Report the Review Board noted

> "In introducing the Voluntary Assisted Dying Bill in 2017, the then Minister for Health stated that the Bill 'balances a compassionate outcome for people at the end of their lives who are suffering and providing community protection' and that the Bill was designed to provide a 'safe and compassionate legislative framework'. Based on the experience of the first 5 years, the Board is satisfied that the objective of safety has been achieved through the Voluntary Assisted Dying Act 2017. However, there are opportunities to enhance the extent to which the goal of providing compassionate care is realised.
>
> The provision of compassionate end of life care, through which the physical and psychological distress that can be associated with dying is minimised, involves person-centred treatment, the promotion of personal autonomy, and an absence of unreasonable or preventable barriers to timely access. The Board considers that these elements can be advanced by adopting some procedural changes in the administration of the Voluntary

Assisted Dying Act 2017 – without diminishing the provisions that have ensured the safe operation of the voluntary assisted dying program to date.

The Board welcomed the Minister's commencement of the Five-Year Review of the Operation of the Voluntary Assisted Dying Act 2017 in 2023. Board members provided their experience and expertise; alongside qualitative and quantitative data collected over the program's operation to support the review process. We extend our thanks to all involved over the past 5 years, and members of the public who contributed to the review. The Board looks forward to the outcome of the review. Further to this, our deliberations on the potential for reviewing the legislation are provided within this report.

Reflections on the reporting year

This reporting period has seen a 22% increase in self-administration permits issued, and a 35% increase in practitioner administration permits. Voluntary assisted dying deaths represented 0.84% of all deaths in Victoria. This compares with 0.65% in the previous reporting year. This is significantly lower than the percentage of voluntary assisted dying deaths in most other States.

The proportion of voluntary assisted dying deaths that involve practitioner administration of the voluntary assisted dying substance in Victoria is 19%. While this an increase on 16% compared to the previous year, it is also significantly lower than in most other States. This reflects the Victorian legislation which requires an applicant be unable to self-administer a substance to be eligible for practitioner administration, versus the right for an applicant to have an element of administration preference in some other jurisdictions.

During the 2023–2024 period, 180 applicants died before being issued a permit, the majority having only completed a First or Consulting assessment before their death. This highlights the ongoing pattern that many patients begin the application process very late in the course of their illness.

Supporting this, just over a quarter (26% of all applications were withdrawn before substance was dispensed (noting that a case can be withdrawn for reasons other than the death of an applicant). Sixty per cent of withdrawn cases were withdrawn because the applicant died less than two weeks after making the first request, representing 15% of all applications.

While those living in rural and regional Victoria can face greater difficulty in accessing voluntary assisted dying, especially given the ban on the use of telehealth, it is notable that while comprising 22% of the Victoria population, rural applicants make up 36% of voluntary assisted dying applicants.

The sustainability of voluntary assisted dying in Victoria

As the offering of voluntary assisted dying as an option for end-of-life care matures in Victoria and we have an opportunity to consolidate the findings of the review, the Board recognises the contributions of medical practitioners to the care and support of Victorians who wish to access voluntary assisted dying.

The Board recognises the ongoing impact of this role. We are concerned about the ongoing sustainability of the program given that the data shows there are only seven medical practitioners trained to provide voluntary assisted dying per 100,000 adults in Victoria.

In 2023–2024, 161 trained medical practitioners coordinated or consulted in at least one application for voluntary assisted dying. Twenty-five per cent of these medical practitioners have only been involved in one case over this reporting year.

Ten doctors with the highest case load over this period either co-ordinated or consulted on 55% of all cases in this 12-month period. Four of these practitioners have been involved in over 50 applications each (of a total 768 applications started) this reporting year.

Of these ten medical practitioners, only three are located in rural and regional Victoria. These 3 practitioners have been involved in 14% of all cases over this period. This level of practitioner engagement has remained consistent since the commencement of the program in June 2019.

The above information highlights that not only does access to voluntary assisted dying rely on a small number of medical practitioners to perform vital duties as co-ordinating or consulting Medical Practitioner, but that this small number of medical practitioners has remained consistent since the commencement of the program.

This is an issue facing all jurisdictions. While the number of medical practitioners registered to provide voluntary assisted dying rose by 14%, a continued focus on widening the training and support for medical practitioners and those who support the process of voluntary assisted dying is important.".

There were 768 applications; 198 were withdrawn; 597 permits were issued; 561 substances were dispensed; 371 VAD deaths occurred. VAD deaths were 0.84% of all deaths in Victoria compared to 0.65% the previous year. The Victoria law allows that if an applicant is unable to self-administer the substance prescribed then they are eligible for the practitioner to administer it. This occurred in 19% of deaths.[27] 180 applicants died before a permit was issued which the report states highlight that patients begin the application process late in the course of their illness. 26% of applications were withdrawn before the substance could be dispensed mostly because the applicant died within 2 weeks of making the first request.

There are 394 medical practitioners with an active profile on the Victoria VAD online portal including 233 General Practitioners, 59 Medical Oncologists, 36 General Physicians, 15 Neurologists and 6 Palliative Medicine specialists.

The Review also highlights that there are constraints on access to VAD because medical practitioners are precluded from initiating a discussion about VAD or to suggest the option; because a person may be reluctant to self-administer the substance; and because there may be limited access to medical practitioners with the experience and specialist qualification required in the law.

South Australia. The South Australian parliament voted a voluntary euthanasia bill into place in 2021 which is similar to the law in Victoria.[22]

New South Wales. In New South Wales, a voluntary Assisted Dying bill was introduced in 2021 and proceeded with amendments to become law in 2022 coming into effect in 2023.[23] A person who wishes assistance with dying who has the capacity to take such a decision voluntarily, can make such a request to a specialist doctor which is then lodged with a Voluntary Assisted Dying Board. The criteria for eligibility are that the person must have a terminal illness that will result in death within 6 months or a neurodegenerative condition that will result in death within 12 months where their suffering is such that it cannot be relieved. Input from a second independent doctor is required with periods for reflection after which the person may be allowed access to a substance to end their life. The substance maybe administered to themselves by the patient, or this may be done by a health practitioner.[23]

Queensland. A voluntary assisted dying act was voted into place by the Queensland Legislative Assembly in 2021 and went into effect in 2023. The eligibility criteria are that their condition must be advanced and progressive with the potential for death within the subsequent 12 months.

People with intact mental capacity who act voluntarily, without coercion and are at least 18 years old may receive assistance in dying.[21]

Tasmania. In Tasmania, the bill referred to as the "End of Life Choices (VAD) Bill" was introduced in 2020 and approved in 2021 coming into effect in 2022. The eligibility criteria are intact decision-making capacity, 18 years of age or older who act voluntarily. They must be suffering intolerably from a medical condition does is incurable, advanced, irreversible and will cause their death within 6 months or 12 months for neurodegenerative disorders. The scheme is subject to stringent regulation.[20]

Western Australia. Western Australian legislators considered a VAD bill in 2019. It passed both the Legislative Council and the Legislative Assembly. Eligibility Required decision taking capacity and 18 years of age and that the person would be terminally ill with a condition causing intolerable suffering likely to cause death within 6 months, or 12 months for a neurodegenerative condition. The support of two independent doctors with both verbal and written requests is required. Self-administration of the lethal medication is permitted but a patient can choose for a medical practitioner to administer the drug.[19]

Australian Capital Territory. ACT governments had indicated a wish to develop AD schemes for some time, but legislation was only possible after a federal legislative ban on AD was lifted. Following a period of consultation and an expert report, a VAD bill 2023 was introduced to the Legislative Assembly. A person 18 years of age or older with intact decision-making capability may apply for assistance in dying if they have an advanced progressive condition. It was passed in 2024 and requires multiple requests and assessment stages by two qualified health professionals. The Capital Territory bill allows assessment by a nurse practitioner. The scheme differs from other states in that those who are eligible do not need to have a specific timeframe until they are expected to die.[24]

Northern Territory. The process of legislation is ongoing and required that the federal government repeal the ban on euthanasia legislation in Australian Territories. After consultation and a report by an expert advisory panel, the recommendation for the introduction of a voluntary assisted dying scheme was accepted and the incoming territorial government is committed to tabling such a bill after further consultation.[25]

What can we learn from the Australian experience so far?

Waller et al.[17] noted "*The 'Australian model' of VAD is highly prescriptive and includes narrow eligibility requirements, a highly regulated request and assessment process, pre-authorisation before administration of VAD in four states, and contemporaneous reporting throughout the process. However, in light of the early Victorian experience, some state laws have significantly departed from the Victorian model: notably introducing more flexible eligibility criteria, different criteria to choose practitioner administration of VAD, and provisions regulating non- participation by facilities*". There are differences in the eligibility criteria including the timeframe used to define Terminal illness (6 months in most States; 12 months in 1 State; a selective 12-month timeframe for neuro degenerative diseases in most States). The NSW and WA Acts require the timeframe to be assessed "on the balance of probabilities". The experience brings attention to the importance of a clear framework of primary legislation and prior reconciliation of federal and state/territorial law. Eligibility criteria are narrow and clear with timelines used to define eligibility. However, there is flexibility to the timelines to reflect the requirements of patients with neurodegenerative diseases in most States. The recognition of the option for clinical assessments by healthcare professionals other than doctors is important. Implementation periods to ensure that the healthcare systems and staff are prepared and trained are required.

Komesaroff and Philip[28] took an overview of the experience in Victoria over 4 years. Their comment that *"there have been no indications of dire consequences either for medicine or for society"* is to be welcomed. They suggest that *"the report card is mixed"* with a system that is respected and functions, usually, smoothly. There has been a steady increase in the numbers of people accessing VAD in Victoria from 179 in year 1 to 443 in year 4. With about one third of the people given a permit, taking the option of VAD (129–306 over the period (we give more details above). 76% of patients have cancer; 9% neurological disease which are very similar to figures in other older permissive jurisdictions, and the largest age group is 70–79, also very similar to other places.81% access palliative care services for a median of 3 months before death. Time from first request to prescription is a median of 34 days, which they feel may be too long for some patients. The workforce pressures mentioned in the 2023–2024 Report[27] are well recognised and patients are often guided through the process by not their usual doctors which is probably not ideal. They confirm the comments made in the Report[27] that preventing HCPs from initiating discussions about VAD is a significant barrier, as was also found in New Zealand. Existing laws have blocked the use of telemedicine - a significant issue for Victoria's widely spread population. Time consuming bureaucracy is an issue and there may be a lack of clarity about how conscientious objections from individuals and institution should operate. There is no evidence that families are suffering an excess of grief or bereavement trauma compared to natural deaths. There is no evidence that VAD has been chosen as an alternative to palliative care, and most patients access both. However, both services are under heavy workload pressure.

In Victoria, this theme of heavy workload pressure on healthcare professionals emerged in a study by Haining et al.[29] who interviewed 37 people engaged in steering and guiding behaviours in VAD on sustaining the workforce. The challenging environment is met with only limited support systems for the HCPs involved and both improvements to existing support systems and new approaches were recommended. The same research team[30] in 2025 explored how HCPs can influence regulation of VAD "at the coalface" and concluded that they can make an influential contribution to the regulatory environment for safe and effective VAD. Molenaar et al.[31] in Victoria examined the impact of VAD on their Palliative Care Service. Only 4% of their clients base expressed interest in VAD and only 1% died through VAD. Early data suggest that a higher proportion of their patients who accessed VAD died in the place of choice in the community than those who did not access VAD.[31] Willmott et al. reported the successful deliver of online training in Victoria.[32]

Komesaroff and Philip[33] and Light et al.[34] in 2024 delivered and commented on surveys of New South Wales (NSW) clinicians following the introduction of VAD. 3010 clinical staff were surveyed and 86% were aware of the new VAD legislation and 76% supportive. Nurses and allied health professionals were more like to be supportive than doctors and only 41% of doctors were willing to take a coordinating role and 23% to administer medications. Michael et al.[35] in NSW reported a mixed impact of VAD enquiries on the quality of Palliative care and the clinical team and emphasise the need for careful prospective studies in this area.

Quite similar results were found in Queensland[36] with 71% of doctors supporting VAD but only 29% being willing to take a coordinating role. Ley et al.[37] in Queensland explored the reasons driving non-participation in interviews with 31 doctors. They identified personal burdens, professional ramifications, external constraints and a reluctance to depart from a traditional medical role, as the main negative factors. Providing continued care, a support for VAD in principle, providing a "good death" and the and the scope of the provision were drivers of a positive attitude to participation. White et al.[38] in Queensland surveyed 24 participants involved VAD delivery in Queensland's Health and Hospital Service. The Service has been largely successful in ensuring patient access to VAD but under resourcing remains a challenge. They note more involvement of nurse practitioners than in other Australian States so far.

Forgione et al.[39] surveyed medical oncologists in South Australia with rather similar results to other States with only 39% willing to participate and 22% conscientious objection. The main barriers to participation were not, however, ethical but they were logistical relating to work pressures and lack of time.

Willmott et al.[40] conducted an early review of Western Australia's VAD Act which came into effect in 2021. Overall, they concluded that the system was working well but with remaining issues to be addressed including awareness of VAD, navigating the system, and workforce. Lamda et al.[41] surveyed 223 doctors and nurses in Western Australia and Victoria a finding, again, that barriers to participation were inadequate remuneration, lack of support and barriers to training access.[41]

Overview

New Zealand and the Australian States have introduced healthcare systems to deliver, monitor, scrutinise and report of AD which are very similar in their eligibility criteria to those proposed in the UK. They have followed cautions legislative and public opinion assessments. Their experience which in one state is for over 5 years, is highly relevant and informative for the UK. Their monitoring and reporting provide us with a rich source of experience upon which the UK and the British Isles can draw. Essentially, the experience in New Zealand and Australia provides a template for the development and implementation of AD legislation, with up to 5 years' experience and monitoring to guide improvements and updating. They are considering modification to some aspects of the procedures and regulation which we can consider prior to the possible implementation in the UK.

The reports of their progress are generally positive and respected and functional systems have been put in place and uptake is as expected in terms of numbers and the diagnoses of people accessing AD. Compliance with regulation has been closely monitored and the rules have been followed with very few exceptions. There is, however, no room for complacency and room for improvements. Clarifications of some aspects of the procedures are needed and some changes in the regulations, notably the barrier to HCPs initiating discussions about AD, may well be changed. Surveys report ongoing pressures on healthcare professionals and workforce challenges.

Experience in New Zealand and the Australian States is probably the best natural comparison for the UK and the British Isles to follow, learn from and improve on, of any of the jurisdictions which permit AD.

References

New Zealand

1. End of Life Choice Act 2019 New Zealand. https://www.legislation.govt.nz/act/public/2019/0067/latest/DLM7285968.html

2. Assisted dying eligibility and access, the eligibility criteria for assisted dying and how to access the service. https://www.tewhatuora.govt.nz/health-services-and-programmes/assisted-dying-service/assisted-dying-information-for-the-public/assisted-dying-eligibility-and-access

3. The Support and Consultation for End of Life in New Zealand (SCENZ) Group. https://www.health.govt.nz/regulation-legislation/assisted-dying/statutory-roles-and-groups/scenz-group

4. Assisted Dying Service yearly report 2021/2022. https://www.tewhatuora.govt.nz/assets/For-the-health-sector/Assisted-Dying/Reporting/assisted-dying-1-year-report-2023-26apr23.pdf

5. Assisted Dying Service Data and Reporting Assisted Dying Service yearly report 2022/2023. https://www.tewhatuora.govt.nz/assets/Health-services-and-programmes/Assisted-Dying-Service/FINAL-assisted-dying-annual-service-report-Nov-2022-Dec-2023.pdf

6. Ngā Ratonga Mate Whakaahuru. Assisted Dying Service Registrar (assisted dying) Annual Report to the Minister of Health. June 2024. https://www.health.govt.nz/system/files/2024-08/registrar_assisted_dying_annual_report_online_version_with_cover_v3.pdf

7. Review of the End of Life Choice Act 2019. https://www.health.govt.nz/system/files/2024-11/review-end-life-choice-act-2019-nov24.pdf

8. Dehkhoda A, Frey R, Carey M, et al. Early experiences of the End-of-Life Choice Act 2019 amongst assisted dying practitioners in Aotearoa New Zealand. BMC Palliative Care, 2025;24:149.

9. Dehkhoda A, Frey R, Carey M, et al. Exploring the impact of e-learning modules and webinars on health professionals' understanding of the End-of-Life Choice Act 2019: a secondary analysis of Manatū Hauora – Ministry of Health workforce survey. N Z Med J. 2023;136(1582):52–63.

10. Snelling J, Young J, Beaumont S, et al. Health care providers' early experiences of assisted dying in Aotearoa New Zealand: an evolving clinical service. BMC Palliat Care. 2023;22(1):101.

11. Sellars M, White BP, Yates P, et al. Medical practitioners' views and experiences of being involved in assisted dying in Victoria, Australia: a qualitative interview study among participating doctors. Soc Sci Med. 2022;292:114568.

12. Wiebe E, Green S, Wiebe K. Medical assistance in dying (MAiD) in Canada: practical aspects for healthcare teams. Ann Palliat Med. 2020;9(6):38–38.

13. Auret K, Pikora TJ, Gersbach K, et al. "Respecting our patients' choices": making the organizational decision to participate in voluntary assisted dying provision: findings from semi-structured interviews with a rural community hospice board of management. BMC Palliat Care. 2022;21(1):1–10.

14. Blaschke S, Schoield P, Taylor K, et al. A. Common dedication to facilitating good dying experiences: qualitative study of end-of-life care professionals' attitudes towards voluntary assisted dying. Palliat Med. 2019;30(6):562–569.

15. Bustin H, Jamieson I, Seay C, et al. A meta-synthesis exploring nurses' experiences of assisted dying and participation decision-making. J Clin Nurs. 2024;33(2):710–723.

16. Mooney N, McCann CM, Tippett L, et al. Decision-making capacity assessments in New Zealand and Australia: a systematised review. Psychiatr Psychol Law. 2023;31(5):816–841.

Australia

17. Waller K, Del Villar K, Willmott L, et al. Voluntary assisted dying in Australia: a comparative and critical analysis of state laws. Univ New South Wales Law J. 2023;46(4):1421–1470.

18. Voluntary Assisted Dying Act 2017 Victoria. https://content.legislation.vic.gov.au/sites/default/files/2020-06/17-61aa004%20authorised.pdf

19. Voluntary Assisted Dying Act 2019 Western Australia. https://www.legislation.wa.gov.au/legislation/prod/filestore.nsf/FileURL/mrdoc_42491.pdf/$FILE/Voluntary%20Assisted%20Dying%20Act%202019%20-%20%5B00-00-00%5D.pdf?OpenElement

20. End-of-Life Choices (Voluntary Assisted Dying) Act 2021 Tasmania. https://www.legislation.tas.gov.au/view/whole/html/asmade/act-2021-001

21. Voluntary Assisted Dying Act 2021 Queensland. https://www.legislation.qld.gov.au/view/pdf/asmade/act-2021-017

22. Voluntary Assisted Dying Act 2021 South Australia. https://www.legislation.sa.gov.au/__legislation/lz/c/a/voluntary%20assisted%20dying%20act%202021/current/2021.29.auth.pdf

23. Voluntary Assisted Dying Act 2022 New South Wales. https://legislation.nsw.gov.au/view/whole/html/inforce/current/act-2022-017#:~:text=An%20Act%20to%20provide%20for,consequential%20amendments%20to%20other%20Acts

24. Voluntary assisted dying in the ACT. https://www.act.gov.au/health/topics/end-of-life-and-palliative-care/voluntary-assisted-dying-in-the-act#:~:text=Voluntary%20assisted%20dying%20will%20be,for%20you%20or%20your%20family

25. Voluntary assisted dying (VAD) in the Northern Territory. https://haveyoursay.nt.gov.au/vad

26. About voluntary assisted dying Overview of eligibility, supports and safeguards. https://www.health.vic.gov.au/voluntary-assisted-dying/about

27. Victoria Voluntary Assisted Dying Review Board July 2023 to June 2024. https://www.health.vic.gov.au/voluntary-assisted-dying/voluntary-assisted-dying-review-board

28. Komesaroff PA, Philip J. Voluntary assisted dying in Victoria: the report card is mixed but we now know what we have to do. Internal Med J 2023;53:2159-2161.

29. Haining CM, Willmott L, White BP. Sustaining the workforce: a qualitative study exploring voluntary assisted dying supports and self-care. Intern Med J. 2025;55(6):1001–1012.

30. Haining CM, Willmott L, White BP. Regulating voluntary assisted dying at the clinical coalface: a qualitative interview study in Victoria, Australia. BMJ Qual Saf. 2025:bmjqs-2024-018314.

31. Molenaar R, Lee S, Lynch J, et al. Voluntary assisted dying and community palliative care: a retrospective study in Victoria, Australia. Nurs Rep. 2025;15(2):34.

32. Willmott L, Feeney R, Yates P AM, et al. A cross-sectional study of the first two years of mandatory training for doctors participating in voluntary assisted dying. Palliat Support Care. 2024;22(4):674–680.

33. Komesaroff PA, Philip J. Clinician attitudes to voluntary assisted dying: what do surveys tell us? Intern Med J. 2024;54(5):703–704.

34. Light E, Kerridge I, Skowronski G, et al. Clinician perspectives on voluntary assisted dying and willingness to be involved: a multisite, cross-sectional survey during implementation in New South Wales, Australia. Intern Med J. 2024;54(5):724–734.

35. Michael N, Jones D, Kernick L, et al. Does voluntary assisted dying impact quality palliative care? A retrospective mixed-method study. BMJ Support Palliat Care. 2024:spcare-2024-004946.

36. Orth C, Henshaw D, Newman W. Doctors' attitudes to voluntary assisted dying in Queensland, Australia. Intern Med J. 2023;53(2):298–299.

37. Ley Greaves L, Willmott L, Feeney R, et al. Assisted dying: participation barriers and facilitators – qualitative interview study of doctors' perceptions. BMJ Support Palliat Care. 2024: spcare-2024-004985.

38. White BP, Ward A, Feeney R, et al. Models of care for voluntary assisted dying: a qualitative study of Queensland's approach in its first year of operation. Aust Health Rev. 2024;48(6):693–699.

39. Forgione MO, Smith A, Hocking CM. Medical oncologist perceptions and willingness to participate in voluntary assisted dying in South Australia. Intern Med J. 2024;54(7):1219–1222.

40. Willmott L, White BP, Haining CM. Review of the Voluntary Assisted Dying Act 2019 (WA): research report. J Law Med. 2025;32(1):94–160.

41. Lamba GT, La Brooy C, Lewis S, et al. Voluntary assisted dying impacts on health professionals. Aust Health Rev. 2024;48(6):720–728.

Chapter 7: International Assisted Dying Laws and Practice: Overview

In Chapters 4–6, we have reviewed the International Experience in AD from the jurisdictions that have legislated to permit AD. There is an extensive and diverse literature, and, in this Chapter, we will bring together an overview of

- The collected Global Statistics of the delivery of AD
- The global literature on Public and Professional attitudes to AD
- International experience of Healthcare Professionals
- International experience of the impact of AD on Healthcare Institutions and Systems
- The literature on the Health Economics of AD

In Chapter 8, we will take an overview of the cultural, religious, disability and disadvantaged people aspects of AD. Chapter 9 will address what we know about patients' and family/ informal caregivers' experience.

The global statistics and practice

In Chapter 4 we noted the overall picture of AD across the world.[1]

- Legislation to permit AD based on intolerable suffering is in place in Canada, Spain, Portugal, Luxembourg, Belgium, the Netherlands, Austria and Switzerland.
- Legislation to permit AD based on established terminal illness usually with a specified period of life expectancy of 6 or 12 months, is in place in the United States, (Washington, Oregon, Hawaii, California, Colorado, New Mexico, Maine, Vermont, New Jersey and the District of Columbia), Australia (South Australia, Western Australia, Queensland, Victoria, Tasmania, NSW) and in New Zealand.
- There is partially permissive legislation in Columbia, Montana, Germany and Italy.

Heidinger et al.[2] (see Chapter 4 for more detail) summarised the global statistics with analysis of 184,695 AD deaths and a total of 12,933,459 deaths (1999–2023). In the most recently reported time periods, the average proportion of deaths (33,088 AD deaths in 1,675,961 total deaths) was 2% ranging from 0.1% in New Jersey to 5.1% in The Netherlands. Over all the jurisdictions, cancer and Motor Neurone Disease account for about 75% of AD deaths, while they account for about 30% of overall deaths. Jurisdictions that permitted only patient self-administration of medications for AD and those that required an estimate of life expectancy had an approximately two-fold lower rates of AD as a proportion of all deaths, than those that permitted healthcare professionals to administer medications or required no estimate of life expectancy. powerful predictor.

Downar et al.[3] have reviewed the international experience for important concerns around eligibility, safeguards, conscientious objection, oversight and reporting for AD. They summarise the international experience in order to explore how to find the best possible balance between safety for patients and access to AD schemes. Key points include:

- All jurisdictions require the patients are capable and fully informed and many require patients to be diagnosed with a terminal illness with an estimated expected lifetime off between 6 and 12 months. Canada, Belgium, Luxembourg and the Netherlands do not specify an expected time frame to death.

- Some countries permit AD for illnesses that are not specified as terminal, but such deaths are relatively uncommon.
- Most assisted deaths globally are for patients with advanced cancer or neurodegenerative disease.
- Safeguards including independent assessment of eligibility, are required, usually with a required pause between the request and the provision of AD.
- Full information about other means of relieving their symptoms, principally palliative care, are usually required and most people who have an assisted death have received palliative care.
- Some jurisdictions prohibit clinicians from initiating conversation about AD, which can restrict access to services.
- In most jurisdictions clinicians may choose not to participate in AD although many do require a referral of the patient to someone who is willing to provide such a service.
- Assisted deaths are usually reviewed by committee retrospectively. Prospective review is used in several jurisdictions to identify ineligible patients.
- Data publication and compliance with safeguards are usual and safeguard violations are rare.
- Concerns that vulnerable people may be coerced into an assisted death are widespread. Studies to evaluate this concern are difficult. Objective measures of vulnerability such as low income, limited education or residence in an institution are associated with a lower likelihood of receiving AD than those who do not have these vulnerabilities.
- Concerns that patients may access AD because they feel they are a burden to their families, or the healthcare system are also widespread. Data from Canada shows that 35% of patients who received AD were reported as feeling that they were a burden. However, patients with advanced cancer who are not pursuing AD, report an even higher prevalence of the perception that they are a burden on their families or the healthcare system, so it is not clear that AD is accessed by people solely for this reason.
- Research into the operation of AD systems and appropriate safeguards is important and essential. This is a challenging field of inquiry

The global literature on public and professional attitudes to AD

Grove et al.[4] published a systematic review of the global literature from 1975 up to July 2023 which addressed quantified support for euthanasia and physician assisted suicide (EAS/AD) among the general public, doctors in various specialties, and nurses. Their review identified 521 studies with 1862 survey questions and 1,945,945 individual responses. The huge dataset allowed powerful meta-analyses of questions relating to public vs professional attitudes, support for different eligibility criteria, different administration protocols, the views of different medical specialties, changes over time and the influence of cultural religious and ethnicity factors. Their conclusions included:

- Doctors were less supportive of EAS/AD than the general public or patients when studies were averaged over this time period (25% vs 55%).

- Nurses were more supportive of EAS than doctors.
- Public support has increased steadily throughout this period from some 40% to some 60% overall support, and public support is greater for AD which has terminal illness, physical illness or severe pain and adulthood as core eligibility requirements than for other criteria.
- Doctors with involvement in caring for terminally ill people were less supportive than those without such involvement.

Table A: USA

State	Legislation	Date	Estimated Life Expectancy for Eligibility for AD
California	End-of-Life Option Act	2015	<6 months
Colorado	End-of-Life Options Act	2016	<6 months
District of Columbia	DC Death with Dignity Act	2016	<6 months
Hawaii	Our Care, Our Choice Act	2018	<6 months
Maine	Death with Dignity Act	2019	<6 months
Montana	Supreme Court ruling in Baxter v Montana	2009	No legal regulations
New Jersey	Medical aid in Dying for the Terminally Ill Act	2019	<6 months
New Mexico	Elizabeth Whitefield End-of-Life Options Act	2021	<6 months
Oregon	Death with Dignity Act	1994	<6 months
Vermont	Patient Choices and Control at End-of-Life Act	2013	<6 months
Washington	Death with Dignity Act	2018	<6 months

Table B: COMMONWEALTH

Country or State	Legislation	Date	Key Eligibility Criteria
Aust. Capital Territory (ACT)	Voluntary Assisted Dying Act in the ACT	2024	Advanced Progressive disease but no specific life expectancy criteria
Canada	An Act to amend the Criminal Code (MAiD)	2016	Enduring and intolerable suffering with reasonably foreseeable death.
		2020	Updated to include option where death is not reasonably foreseeable
New South Wales	Voluntary Assisted Dying Act New South Wales	2022	Incurable, advanced and progressive disease with death expected within 6 months or 12 months for neurodegenerative disease
New Zealand	End of Life Choice Act	2019	Terminal illness likely to end life within 6 months
Northern Territory	Pending	Pending	Pending

Country or State	Legislation	Date	Key Eligibility Criteria
Queensland	Voluntary Assisted Dying Act Queensland	2021	Incurable, advanced and progressive disease with death expected within 12 months
South Australia	Voluntary Assisted Dying Act South Australia	2021	Incurable, advanced and progressive disease with death expected within 6 months or 12 months for neurodegenerative disease
Tasmania	End-of-Life Choices Voluntary Assisted Dying Act Tasmania	2021	Incurable, advanced and progressive disease with death expected within 6 months or 12 months for neurodegenerative disease
Victoria Au	Voluntary Assisted Dying Act Victoria	2017	Incurable, advanced and progressive disease with death expected within 6 months or 12 months for neurodegenerative disease
Western Australia	Voluntary Assisted Dying Act Western Australia	2019	Incurable, advanced and progressive disease with death expected within 6 months or 12 months for neurodegenerative disease

Table C: EUROPE

Country or State	Legislation	Date	Eligibility Criteria
Austria	Will to Die Law	2022	Severe, permanent illness affecting entire life
Belgium	Belgian Act on Euthanasia	2002	Medically hopeless condition, suffering unbearably, serious disorder without remedy
France	End of Life Bill	Pending	Serious and incurable disease, life-threatening and in its advanced or terminal phases
Germany	Ruling of the Constitutional Court	2020	The freedom to take one's own life also encompasses the freedom to seek and make use of assistance by third parties
Ireland	Dignity with Dying	Pending	Pending
Italy	Ruling of the Constitutional Court 242 ruling	2019	No specific criteria
Luxembourg	Law on the Right to Die with Dignity	2009	Unbearable physical or psychological suffering due to an incurable illness
Netherlands	Termination of Life on Request and Assisted Suicide (Review Procedures) Act	2002	Suffering is unbearable, with no prospect of improvement, no reasonable alternative
Portugal	Medically assisted death is not punishable and amends the Penal Code	2023 (pending)	Terminally ill or suffering from a serious and incurable illness or injury, and experiencing intense, lasting, and unbearable suffering
Spain	Law Regulating Euthanasia	2021	Severe, chronic, debilitating, or incurable disease

International experience of healthcare professionals

The experience and attitudes of healthcare professionals (HCPs) who work in jurisdictions which permit AD will be of considerable value to those in other countries where new legislation is being considered or enacted. Understandably there is a considerable amount of work and interest in this area with several reports, studies and reviews summarising and analysing the experiences, emotional responses and reflections of HCPs involved with AD provision. We are unable to provide a systematic review in this chapter but seek to give an overview of the main themes and learning. More details of the experiences in AD jurisdictions are given in Chapters 4-6.

Medicine is rooted in the ethical principle of 'first, do no harm'. AD can be seen to challenge this traditional and basic principle. Set against this backdrop is the loss of control, distress and symptoms experienced by some patients at the end of life which can lead to a sense of moral ambiguity and tension for healthcare professionals. Moral distress is defined as "...when one knows the right thing to do, but institutional constraints make it nearly impossible to pursue the right course of action."[5] There is conflicting evidence about whether HCPs involved in AD experience moral distress and to what level, with many physicians reporting a great deal of satisfaction and gratification being involved in the AD process.[6-9] Many HCPs report a great pride in deliver of a 'good death', a sense of fulfilment and satisfaction associated with providing and delivering patient choice at the end of life. However, others report emotional burden or discomfort that could lead to ongoing adverse impact.

Researchers from Canada[10] attempted to answer the question, 'what it means at an emotional level', for a healthcare practitioner involved with AD. Data from 35 studies (393 physicians, 169 nurses, 53 social workers, 22 allied healthcare professionals) from five countries were analysed. Diverse research methods were noted but thematic meta-synthesis showed three descriptive emotional themes. Firstly strong, polarised emotions, both positive (reward, relief, openness) and negative (guild, emotional exhaustion) but also moral distress or 'shudder' shaped by cultural and political factors. Secondly, reflective emotions with AD as a 'sense-making process' involving deeper processing such as 'growing through patient experiences and challenging death taboos. And thirdly, emotions resonating with professional values linking to themes such as competency and 'intimate care'.

Two overarching analytical insights were described to postulate why HCPs experienced complex emotions. The legislative framework around AD affected HCP emotional impact. In countries where AD is tied to terminal illness (the USA, New Zealand, Australia), HCPs show more polarised emotions, influenced by cultural and personal beliefs. In contrast, where AD is allowed for non-terminal suffering (e.g. Switzerland, Belgium, the Netherlands) AD was seen as a reflective, philosophical process, helping HCPs reconcile internal emotional conflict. The second factor was the values associated with the profession and engagement with AD. Nurses, due to their close patient contact and caregiving ethos, often experience intense emotional reactions, both positive (fulfilment) and negative (burden, distress).

A more recent review from Pinto[11] reviewed 30 studies from 2017 to 2023 for the perceived risks, harms, and benefits to doctors of administering AD (E/PS euthanasia/Physician-assisted suicide) They highlight 5 themes from the synthesis of qualitative studies: (i) experience of the request prior to administration which varied from feelings of being helpful to the patient at EOL to intense moral distress and conflict; (ii) the doctor's role and agency in the death of a patient creating tension between the autonomy of the doctor and patient; (iii) moral distress post-administration with clear dichotomy of views expressed in studies; (iv) increased workload and burnout experienced by HCPS engaged in AD and (v) the importance of professional guidance and support.

They conclude: "*These findings showcase the complexity of E/PS for participating clinicians, high-lighting the need for further research into the impact of administering E/PS on doctors specifically focusing on moral injury; better support structures for doctors post-administration; greater funding and strategies to improve palliative care for patients who seek E/PAS due to a sense of demoralisation; and how to understand why some doctors are negatively emotionally affected by involvement in E/PAS, while others can feel fulfilled by similar actions. How do we adequately support clinicians to navigate this challenging area?*". How indeed? It's crucial that the psychological wellbeing of HCPs involved in AD is addressed, researched and supported in the UK if AD becomes legal.

Komesaroff and Philip[12,13] reported on the first four years of experience of AD in Victoria, Australia and noted a steady increase in the number of cases from 179 in 2019 to 443 in 2023. As expected most common diagnosis was cancer 76% and neurological diseases accounted for 9%. 81% of patients had accessed palliative care services prior to death. A number of challenges to HCPs were reported. The Victoria Act prevented doctors from introducing the possibility of AD and this had been found to inhibit communication and limitations on telemedical consultations. There were concerns about time delays and shortages of trained practitioners. Many doctors reported pressure on the time available for AD discussions and completing required paperwork, with note made of lack of financial compensation for this work. Furthermore, they draw attention to the fact that the effects on other health providers is uncertain, and that few formal systems of support have been developed by health services for their staff. For patients there was reassurance that there were no differences in bereavement outcomes for those accessing AD or those who did not do so. There was no evidence the patients had chosen AD as an alternative to palliative care. The authors emphasise the importance of constant monitoring of the process and the impact of AD and the updating of procedures to reflect new knowledge and understanding.

Komesaroff and Philip[12] and Sellars et al.[14] reported on surveys of clinician attitudes in Australia following the introduction of AD. They report widespread support for AD among clinicians and the general increase in support over time. However, only a small proportion of practitioners are prepared to become directly involved.

Other studies from Australia assess the physician reported barriers to participation in AD. Greaves et al.[15] report on 31 doctors from Queensland who had no in-principle objection. The barriers were personal burdens, professional ramifications and potential stigma, external/resource constraints and the difference from the traditional role of a doctor. The facilitators to participation included the provision of continuation of care, philosophical support for AD, ability to provide a good death and the scope of provision. And these results are consistent with a further Queensland based study by Lamba et al.[16] who surveyed 223 healthcare professionals to assess the impact of AD procedures. The barriers identified were inadequate remuneration, a need for professional support and difficulties accessing training.

Similarly, Forgione et al.[17] surveyed 67 South Australian medical oncologists and found that 39% reported willingness to participate in AD and 22% reported a conscientious objection to participation. Of those without a conscientious objection, the main barriers to participation were lack of time and lack of training. It's clear some of these barriers are modifiable.

Willmott et al.[18] studied the first two years of mandatory training for 289 doctors participating in AD In Victoria. Almost all participants found the training to be helpful or very helpful and became confident in their knowledge and application of the VAD legislation. This highlights the need for AD specific training for clinicians involved in the services.

In summary, there are a range of complex emotions experienced by HCPs involved in the AD process with can be shaped by legal context, personal conscience, and professional values. Whilst many clinicians report positive emotions associated with the provision of AD, any jurisdiction allowing AD needs to be mindful of the emotional pressure and potential negative impact and distress that this service can cause amongst some. Furthermore, it is clear from recent experience in both Canada and Australia that streamlined practical processes are important to aid those HCPs involved in AD services navigate the system with the need for dedicated training, time and support for all.

International experience of the impact of AD on healthcare institutions and systems

Hewitt et al.[19] conducted an integrative review of 58 studies addressing the factors that influence access the health services for AD across Canada, the USA, the Netherlands, Australia, Belgium and New Zealand with the views of 8503 stakeholders, published between 1998 and 2024. They used a framework developed by Levesque et al.,[20] which characterises the "supply-side" dimensions which reflect what is expected of the healthcare provider services and the "demand-side" as the abilities of potential patients and carers to access those services. Supply-side dimensions used are approachability, acceptability, availability and accommodation, affordability and appropriateness. "Demand side" abilities include the patients' needs, health literacy, health beliefs, trust in healthcare, personal and social values, culture, autonomy, transport, mobility, social support, income, assets, insurance, social capital (community support) empowerment and caregiver support.[20]

Supply-side dimensions were

- *Approachability.* Hewitt et al.[20] report that healthcare institutions are available in their degree of transparency to the provision of AD services and there is a need for approaches to ensure patients can readily identify which institutions are available to them. This may be tackled by individual institutions or system wide information sources.[21–24]

- *Acceptability.* Access to AD services may be influenced by the views of healthcare professional who may have conscience based or work-pressure based reservations[25–28] or the reservations of healthcare institutions. Hospices may have institutional values and/or constitutions which preclude them from participating in AD and this will shape access and the service available.[29–31]

- *Availability.* Rural and remote communities may rely on telemedicine for eligibility assessments[32] but procedural, resource and staffing barriers may apply in any setting.[33–36]

- *Affordability* for HCPs and their institutions is an issue with reports that remuneration may not match the time required and that the pressure of delivering AD can be intense.[34,37–39]

- *Appropriateness* in the Levesque framework refers to the clinicians' ability to evaluate the patients' needs accurately which requires experience and training for the HCPs involved and support from their institutions.[40]

"Demand side" abilities which determine a patients approach to accessing AD services in the Levesque framework were lists above (the patients' needs, health literacy, health beliefs, trust in healthcare, personal and social values, culture, autonomy, transport, mobility, social support, income, assets, insurance, social capital (community support) empowerment, and caregiver support).[20]

Brooke Russell et al.[41] used patient reported outcome measures to evaluate the symptom burdens of patients who accessed MAiD in Canada and compared them to those who did not do so. Although MAiD patients had greater symptom burdens in some domains (anxiety and loss of appetite) the reported differences between the two groups were not large. Patients' reasons for seeking AD were influenced by their wish for autonomy and dignity, fear of increasing severity of symptoms, dependency, loss of a sense of self and a need to control the manner of their death.[20] Immobility can restrict access to AD[32,42] and cost to the patient is an issue in some jurisdictions.[20]

Worthington et al.[43] reviewed recent literature on the delivery of AD and suggested a comprehensive list of the challenges faced by institutions which set up AD services.

Health economic analysis

The implications of AD for the cost of healthcare services have been substantially discussed. Those who support and those who oppose the introduction of legislation permitting AD have commented on its potential to alter the costs of healthcare for those at the end of life. There is very little healthcare data and research which allows an objective evaluation of such costs.

Isaac et al.[44] conducted a rigorous systematic review of available publications. They concluded that there is very little health economic analysis that meets the rigorous standards required to allow reliable conclusions. The absence of such reliable conclusions makes it impossible to make decisions on the introduction of AD based on its impact on healthcare costs. Of the 2790 screened articles, only three met the criteria for inclusion in the review, two from Canada and one from the United States. These three studies all showed that the introduction of AD laws would reduce healthcare spending on end-of-life care. However, their relevance to the other healthcare systems is very uncertain. Hudson et al.[45] attempted to evaluate the cost and resource implications of AD but found a paucity of detail regarding actual costs. Both Canadian and UK Governments have carried out health service cost impact exercises on the in implementation of AD and, within broad ranges of uncertainty, suggest that introducing AD reduces healthcare spending over time.[46,47]

In conclusion, the global statistics and the overviews of the systems and procedures introduced for AD suggest that if societies and their legislators decide that they wish to introduce AD, then it is possible to do so but with great caution and attention to detail.

We discuss the patient and public centred issue in other chapters, but here we must draw attention to the seriousness and scale of the impact of a new AD system on healthcare individuals and institutions. Some will have ethical and religious constraints, and these must be address by allowing conscience driven decisions about their involvement. However, the literature clearly shows that the concerns of healthcare professionals often focus on the workload pressures and logistics.

The available data suggest that AD systems do not add overall cost to the healthcare budgets of jurisdictions which introduce them. So, it should be possible to ensure adequate resources are available. However, most healthcare professional have concerns about the ability of healthcare systems to place resources in the right place at the right time, and they will hope for and need meticulous planning of the delivery of AD procedures to ensure that they are not inadequately planned or resourced. In the UK and often internationally, Palliative Care at the end of life is often under resourced worldwide and practitioners in this discipline are understandably anxious that changes in the law, could have negative impacts on the resources available for their, already hard-pressed, services.

References

1. Looi MK. Assisted dying laws around the world. BMJ. 2024;387:q2385.
2. Heidinger B, Webber C, Chambaere K, et al. International comparison of underlying disease among recipients of medical assistance in dying. JAMA Intern Med. 2025;185(2):235–237.
3. Downar J, Close E, Young JE, et al. Assisted dying: balancing safety with access. BMJ. 2024;387:q2382.

4. Grove GL, Lovell MR, Hughes I, et al. Voluntary-assisted dying, euthanasia and physician-assisted suicide: global perspectives-systematic review. BMJ Support Palliat Care. 2025;15(4):423–435.

5. Jameton, A. Nursing Practice: The Ethical Issues. Prentice-Hall, 1984.

6. Beuthin, R, Bruce, A, Hopwood, M, et al. Rediscovering the art of medicine, rewards, and risks: physicians' experience of providing medical assistance in dying in Canada. SAGE Open Medicine 8, 2020.

7. Wibisono, S, Minto, K, Lizzio-Wilson, M, et al. Attitudes toward and experiences with assisted-death services and psychological implications for health practitioners: a narrative systematic review. Omega (Westport). 2025;91(2):590-612. doi: 10.1177/00302228221138997.

8. Kelly B, Handley T, Kissane D, et al. "An indelible mark" the response to participation in euthanasia and physician-assisted suicide among doctors: a review of research findings. Palliative and Supportive Care. 2020;18(1):82–88.

9. Green S. This is assisted dying. a doctor's story of empowering patients at the end of life. Scribner, March 2022. ISBN: ISBN-13: 978-1668004784.

10. Dholakia SY, Bagheri A, Simpson A. Emotional impact on healthcare providers involved in medical assistance in dying (MAiD): a systematic review and qualitative meta-synthesis. BMJ Open. 2022;12(7):e058523.

11. Pinto P, Fogarty GB, Kissane D. Narrative review of the impact on physicians of administering euthanasia or physician-assisted suicide and its association with moral distress. Palliat Support Care. 2025;23:e115.

12. Komesaroff PA, Philip J. Voluntary assisted dying in Victoria: the report card is mixed but we now know what we have to do. Internal Med J. 2023;53:2159–2161.

13. Komesaroff PA, Philip J. Clinician attitudes to voluntary assisted dying: what do surveys tell us? Intern Med J. 2024;54(5):703–704.

14. Sellars M, White BP, Yates P, et al. Medical practitioners' views and experiences of being involved in assisted dying in Victoria, Australia: a qualitative interview study among participating doctors. Soc Sci Med. 2022;292:114568.

15. Ley Greaves L, Willmott L, Feeney R, et al. Assisted dying: participation barriers and facilitators – qualitative interview study of doctors' perceptions. BMJ Support Palliat Care. 2024:spcare-2024-004985.

16. Lamba GT, La Brooy C, Lewis S, et al. Voluntary assisted dying: impacts on health professionals. Aust Health Rev. 2024;48(6):720–728.

17. Forgione MO, Smith A, Hocking CM. Medical oncologist perceptions and willingness to participate in voluntary assisted dying in South Australia. Intern Med J. 2024;54(7):1219–1222.

18. Willmott L, Feeney R, Yates PAM, et al. A cross-sectional study of the first two years of mandatory training for doctors participating in voluntary assisted dying. Palliat Support Care. 2024;22(4):674–680.

19. Hewitt J, Wilson M, Bonner A, et al. Factors that influence access to medical assistance in dying services: an integrative review. Health Expect. 2024;27(5):e70058.

20. Levesque JF, Harris MF, Russell G. Patient-centred access to health care: conceptualising access at the interface of health systems and populations. Int J Equity Health. 2013;12:18.

21. Thomas R, Pesut B, Puurveen G, et al. Medical assistance in dying: a review of Canadian health authority policy documents. Global Qual Nurs Res. 2023;10: 233339362311673.

22. Silvius JL, Memon A, Arain M. Medical assistance in dying: Alberta approach and policy analysis. Can J Aging. 2019;38(3):397–406.

23. Close E, Willmott L, Keogh, L et al. Institutional objection to voluntary assisted dying in Victoria, Australia: an analysis of publicly available policies. J Bioeth Inq. 2023;20(3):467–484.

24. Sellars M, White BP, Yates P, et al. Medical practitioners' views and experiences of being involved in assisted dying in Victoria, Australia: a qualitative interview study among participating doctors. Soc Sci Med. 2022;292:114568.

25. Brown J, Goodridge D, Thorpe L, et al. "I Am Okay With It, But I Am Not Going to Do It": the exogenous factors influencing non-participation in medical assistance in dying. Qual Health Res. 2021;31(12):2274–2289.

26. Kortes-Miller K, Durant KL. Physician experiences with medical assistance in dying: Qualitative study in northwestern Ontario. Can Fam Physician. 2022;68(5):e161–e168.

27. Campbell EG, Kini V, Ressalam J, et al. Physicians' attitudes and experiences with medical aid in dying in Colorado: a "hidden population" survey. J Gen Intern Med. 2022;37(13):3310–3317.

28. Rutherford J, Willmott L, White BP. What the doctor would prescribe: physician experiences of providing voluntary assisted dying in Australia. Omega (Westport). 2023;87(4):1063–1087.

29. Cain CL, Koenig BA, Starks H, et al. Hospital and health system policies concerning the California End of Life Option Act. J Palliat Med. 2020;23(1):60–66.

30. Campbell CS, Black MA. Dignity, death, and dilemmas: a study of Washington hospices and physician-assisted death. J Pain Symptom Manage. 2014;47(1):137–153.

31. Campbell CS, Cox JC. Hospice-assisted death? A study of Oregon hospices on death with dignity. Am J Hosp Palliat Care. 2012;29(3):227–235.

32. Dion S, Wiebe E, Kelly M. Quality of care with telemedicine for medical assistance in dying eligibility assessments: a mixed-methods study. CMAJ Open. 2019;7(4):E721–E729.

33. Brown J, Goodridge D, Thorpe L, et al. "What is right for me, is not necessarily right for you": the endogenous factors influencing nonparticipation in medical assistance in dying. Qual Health Res. 2021;31(10):1786–1800.

34. de Boer ME, Depla MFIA, den Breejen M, et al. Pressure in dealing with requests for euthanasia or assisted suicide. Experiences of general practitioners. J Med Ethics. 2019;45(7):425–429.

35. White BP. Jeanneret R, Close E, et al. Access to voluntary assisted dying in Victoria: a qualitative study of family caregivers' perceptions of barriers and facilitators. Med J Austr. 2023;219:211–217.

36. Snelling J, Young J, Beaumont S, et al. Health care providers' early experiences of assisted dying in Aotearoa New Zealand: an evolving clinical service. BMC Palliat Care. 2023;22(1):101.

37. Shaw J, Wiebe E, Nuhn A, et al. Providing medical assistance in dying: practice perspectives. Can Fam Physician 2018;64(9):394.

38. Khoshnood N, Hopwood MC, Lokuge B, et al. Exploring Canadian physicians' experiences providing medical assistance in dying: a qualitative study. J Pain Symptom Manag 2018;56(2): 222–229.e1.

39. Gerson SM, Preston NJ, Bingley AF. Medical aid in dying, hastened death, and suicide: a qualitative study of hospice professionals' experiences from Washington state. J Pain Symptom Manage. 2020;59(3):679–686.e1.

40. Ten Cate K, van Tol DG, van de Vathorst S. Considerations on requests for euthanasia or assisted suicide; a qualitative study with Dutch general practitioners. Fam Pract. 2017;34(6):723–729.

41. Russell KB, Forbes C, Qi S, et al. End-of-life symptom burden among patients with cancer who were provided medical assistance in dying (MAID): a longitudinal propensity-score-matched cohort study. Cancers (Basel). 2024;16(7):1294.

42. Fischer S, Huber CA, Furter M, et al. Reasons why people in Switzerland seek assisted suicide: the view of patients and physicians. Swiss Med Wkly. 2009;139(23-24):333–338.

43. Worthington A, Finlay I, Regnard C. Assisted dying and medical practice: questions and considerations for healthcare organisations. BMJ Support Palliat Care. 2023;13(4):438–441.

44. Isaac S, McLachlan AJ, Chaar B. Policies and cost analyses of voluntary assisted dying (VAD) laws – a mapping review & analysis. Health Econ Rev. 2024;14(1):66.

45. Hudson P, Marco D, De Abreu Lourenco R, et al. What are the cost and resource implications of voluntary assisted dying and euthanasia? Aust Health Rev. 2024;48(3):269–273.

46. Terminally Ill Adults (End of Life) Bill: impact assessment (updated). https://assets.publishing.service.gov.uk/media/68247bfdb9226dd8e81ab849/terminally-ill-adults-end-of-life-bill-impact-assessment-updated.pdf

47. Cost estimate for Bill C-7 "Medical Assistance In Dying" 2020. https://qsarchive-archiveqs.pbo-dpb.ca/web/default/files/Documents/Reports/RP-2021-025-M/RP-2021-025-M_en.pdf

Chapter 8: **The Importance of Cultural
and Religious Issues and the Views of
Disadvantaged and/or Disabled People**   81

Chapter 8: The Importance of Cultural and Religious Issues and the Views of Disadvantaged and/or Disabled People

In this chapter we will address the cultural and religious issues which have arisen in the discussions of AD and the international peer reviewed literature that sheds some light on them. We have then addressed the literature on the views of disabled people and the issues around disability, disadvantage and vulnerability which have a central role in the debates about AD and possible changes in the law to permit AD in some jurisdictions and under some circumstances.

Bloomer et al.[1] conducted a scoping review of the academic, peer reviewed, literature in English on the racial, ethnic and cultural perspectives of AD. They searched for studies which included participants who were identified with "culturally diverse tributes including ancestry, country of birth, ethnicity, cultural heritage, language, religion or which were considered different from other groups in the community or society in which they reside or interact" excluding healthcare workers from the study. They identified 17 such studies published between 1993 and 2022.[2-18] They presented their findings in two themes

- *Religious and spiritual perspectives.* Ten studies addressed the perspectives on AD from Muslim, Jewish, Buddhist, Evangelical-Lutheran, Pentecostal and Seventh Day Adventist churches, Hare-Krishna and the Union of Free Thinkers participants including 5 which focussed on religiosity and spirituality.
- *Race, Ethnicity and ancestry.* Ten studies addressed the views of participants from these backgrounds with some variable terminology, but descriptions included African American and Black, Asian (including Chinese, Chinese Australian, Filipino, and Japanese), Caucasian (including Anglo-Australian, Non-Hispanic White, white Californian, Hispanic and native Hawaiian.

Some studies included both themes. The studies reported include a rich, complex and diverse set of perspectives with few simple conclusions. There was diversity within all groups. However, Bloomer et al.[1] do conclude that the influence of religiosity, religious beliefs and spirituality is significant for most interviewed participants and the majority report a negative perception of Assisted Dying with many reporting that it was against their religious beliefs.

There was no consistent pattern across all the race/ethnicity/ancestry groups interviewed with diversity between and within studies.

Bloomer et al concluded:

- *"Religiosity, religious beliefs and spirituality had a clear influence on perceptions of assisted dying, enabling individuals 'clear and unequivocal stance on assisted dying.*
- *Cultural attributes are many and complex, resulting in a spectrum of perspectives on assisted dying, and not all people assumed to have the same cultural attribute will hold the same perspective.*
- *In addition to perspectives of assisted dying linked to cultural attributes, concern for vulnerable or marginalised people, those who lack resources to enable autonomy, and those who fear being a burden were also shared.*

• *Promoting an awareness of, and openness to understanding the relationship between racial, ethnic and cultural attributes and the care provided to people with life-limiting illness, their family and carers across practice settings including palliative care is essential to supporting choice at the end of life".*

We reported in more detail in Chapter 1 that Opinium UK,[19] sponsored by the campaign group Dignity in Dying, which is a supporter of legislation to permit AD, conducted an online survey amongst a sample of 10,897 UK Adults in February 2024,[20] which includes a link to the Excel Spreadsheet). The Net Support result was consistent (over 70%) across the UK Devolved Nations and English regions except London (67%) and Northern Ireland (66%). Other groups whose Net Support scores were below 70% were those declaring themselves to be Religious (66%); all Christians (69%); Catholic (65%); Muslims (34%); Hindu (58%); Jewish (61%); Sikh (62%); Asian people (48%); Black people (47%) and those aged 18–24 years (68%). This suggests that views in the UK generally reflect the international findings.

The thorough scoping review from Bloomer et al.[1] covered the literature up to 2022. We have searched the medical literature on the topics of "Ethnicity" and of "Religion" and AD from 2022 to mid-2025. Kozlov et al.[21] reported on 3227 respondents asked about their knowledge and attitudes. Notably across all US States, those that permit AD and those that do not, only a little over half of the respondents were aware that AD is legal in any jurisdictions in the USA (51.3%), with a slightly higher proportion in States with permissive AD legislation. When asked if they would consider accessing AD for a terminal illness, 44% overall said they would do so, with modest differences among the groups of people surveyed (43% Asian respondents, 34% of Black respondents and 42% of Hispanic respondents). In New Zealand, Asian health professionals were less likely to support AD than European/Pakeha counterparts.[22] Grundig et al.[23] conducted a systematic review of 49 studies of attitudes to end of life care including AD and found that religious belief was a significant factor which was also the case for Canadian and Pakistani undergraduates.[24,25] The impact of religious belief on medical practitioners in the USA[26] was substantial with 26% reporting large ethical or religious barriers to their involvement in AD. The religious affiliation of healthcare institutions resulted in the transfer of 9% of patients to different institutions for AD in Canada during COVID.[27] In countries which do not permit AD religious belief is a significant factor in the attitudes of the public and healthcare professionals, in Japan,[28] Croatia,[29] Lithuania,[30] India[31] and the approach to AD in Spain.[32]

The concerns and views of disabled people

The views of disabled people and the issues surrounding disability and vulnerability and AD in the UK are complex. There is no consensus among disabled peoples' organisations or their professional advisors. Public statements are polarised.[33–38]

Disabled People's Organisations have united in the opposition to the current Bill before the UK Parliament(R). Disability Rights UK[34] says "*At Disability Rights UK, our trustees reviewed our position on assisted dying, moving from being neutral to being against. This shift was heavily influenced by our experience of COVID, where almost 60% of deaths were of Disabled people, alongside active devaluing and de-prioritisation of our lives. Another factor that influenced the change in our position was the continued significant underfunding of public services, in particular social care, which is supposed to give hundreds of thousands of Disabled people the everyday care and support we need to live full and dignified lives. The aim of Disability Rights UK is to create an inclusive society for Disabled people – we don't believe that the Bill moves us in this direction.*"

The key reasons for their opposition to the Bill were given to be that it devalues the lives of Disabled people; perpetuates systemic inequalities; reflects conflicting NHS Cultures; has insufficient safeguards and there has been a poor Parliamentary process. DRUK says "*It feels hugely unjust to have the spotlight put on the right to die, when millions of us are being denied the right to live. Disability Rights UK will continue to work with Not Dead Yet, DPAC, Inclusion London and others to campaign against the Bill, highlighting ableism and inequality, inadequate protections, unsatisfactory Bill process and lack of engagement with Disabled people*".

On the other hand, Trevor Moore, Chair of My Death, My Decision, said[37]:

'*We must of course hear the voices of assisted dying opponents, but conversely, we cannot allow hypothetical concerns to be a disproportionate distraction from the lived reality of countless people whose suffering is protracted while we await a compassionate law. Knowing that they could control the manner and timing of their own death, if and when they so choose, will in itself be of real comfort.*

In the discussion of assisted dying it is crucial that we base decisions on evidence. Regrettably, there are opponents of a law who not only purport to speak for all disabled people but also paint alarming pictures of assisted dying that are simply not borne out by the evidence from countless places that allow it.'

Box and Chambaere[39] collected the then views of Disability Rights Organisations and found the most did not have a clear public position and there was considerable diversity of opinion. Opposed organisations were of the view that legislation to permit AD would be premature misguided, inequitable and culturally undesirable. Those in support of new legislation agued it could promote autonomy and end intense suffering. Reasons given to oppose AD laws included the inadequacy of current Palliative Care services, the risk that Disabled people would be pressured into opting for AD, that there could be a "slippery slope" towards widening the eligibility for AD, and the doctor-patient relationship would be undermined. They concluded that whatever views might prevail in the organisations, it is vital that all their voices are heard, and concerns addressed. We discussed the opinion poll surveys in Chapter 1. The large Opinium poll[19] indicated that people reporting themselves to be Disabled recorded Net Support for AD at 78%.

Lewis reviewed the issue of AD in vulnerable groups in our 2020 book.[40] She concluded that there was no evidence that the legal criteria that apply to an individual's request for AD are not well respected and that the available evidence suggested that the uptake of AD was more likely in groups who appeared to be socially privileged. Battin et al.[41] studied the impact of AD in vulnerable groups and concluded that those who received AD were more likely to enjoy comparative social, economic, educational and professional and other privileges[41] although Lewis notes that the absence of data on preexisting disability in the Oregon data weakens the conclusions about disability. The Battin study[41] has been quoted as showing no evidence of an excess of AD in any group, and for age, gender, medical insurance status the data are robust; for educational status, poverty they are reasonably robust. The data on ethnicity was limited to small numbers. The data on patients receiving AD who had a preexisting disability separate from their terminal illness can only be inferred but does suggest there were few if any patients with preexisting disabilities who received AD unless they also had a serious illness.[41] Rietjens et al.[42] in a systematic review of the peer reviewed literature found that there was no evidence that AD was increased in groups with vulnerability or disability and the only social factor associated with increased uptake was higher education.[42] Steck[43] reviewed the published literature and found more AD uptake in those with higher education and no religious beliefs but not in those who were disabled or vulnerable. Emanuel et al.[44] reviewed the data from multiple jurisdictions with permissive AD legislation and concluded that the suggestion that people with disabilities would be more likely to access AD was not supported by the findings. Dierickx et al.[45] reported the increase in AD uptake in Belgium between 2007 and 2013 but there was no overrepresentation of people with disabilities. Colburn[46] reviewed the literature to date and argued that there is little empirical evidence that patients who are vulnerable or have disabilities are overrepresented in those who access AD.

Redelmeier et al.[47] studied a total of 50,096 palliative care deaths in Ontario between 2016 and 2019, of which 920 received MAiD under universal health insurance, such that there were no direct financial incentives or disincentives to take up MAiD. They conducted extensive statistical case adjustments for potential imbalances. MAiD uptake was commoner among patients with higher socioeconomic status (2.4%) than those with lower such status (1.5%).

We are only aware of one study published since that time which shows empirically an excess of people of low socioeconomic status, who may be perceived to be vulnerable, among those who access AD. Tran et al.[48] in Western Ontario, among 408 requests for MAiD, found a disproportionately high number requests for AD form patients of low socioeconomic status.[48] Canada changed its eligibility criteria for MAiD in 2021 so that these data may not apply precisely to the current status of MAiD. Asada et al.[49] were able to begin to assess the relationship between MAiD for patients who had a Terminal Illness whose death is reasonably foreseeable (called Track 1 in MAiD reports - see Chapter 2) and those in Track 2 whose death is not reasonably foreseeable. It is difficult to evaluate whether reports of disability reflect disability due to a recent illness such as cancer which is causing loss of abilities or a pre-existing longer term disability. However, it was the case that higher levels of disability are reported in the relatively small number of cases of MAiD in Track 2. Asada et al emphasise the importance of prospective complete and accurate data collection to monitor these impacts on future experience.[49] Fully understanding the impacts of disability and disadvantage on the uptake of MAiD requires careful evaluation of the availability of healthcare systems as well as the knowledge and attitudes of patients from a variety of backgrounds and abilities. Asada draws attention to the disparities in access to healthcare systems across Canada geographically and socially.[49] Berube et al.[50] studied knowledge and attitudes to end of life care in Canada. They noted the barriers to access care among those with social or economic disadvantages, and that their knowledge of end-of-life care options was relatively low, but also that there was a positive attitude to MAiD.

The ongoing debates on the relationship between disadvantage and disability have many facets and points of view, including:

- The impact that AD may have on the trust that patients may feel towards their healthcare and advisors. Concerns are that the mention of AD may engender a lack of trust reflecting a fear that healthcare staff may promote AD as an inappropriate solution for patients with terminal illness or chronic severe illness. These concerns are widely felt. Anderson et al.[51] somewhat unusually in this field, used a randomised survey approach to test this concern using a formal measurement instrument for patients trust. They randomised patients who reported being unaware that MAiD was legal in in their jurisdiction, either to receive notification that MAiD is legal or to receive no such notification. Those who were told MAiD was legal were more likely to approve of its use, but they showed no significant differences in measures of trust in healthcare professionals.

- In jurisdictions where only self-administration of medication for AD is permitted, this is seen to disadvantage people who have disabilities which prevent them taking their medication by themselves.[52-54]

- Hopkins et al.[55] drew attention to the importance of considering the implications of AD for frail, often elderly people. This clinical group may not be regarded traditionally as having a terminal illness, their prognosis may be difficult relatively to predict and treatment to relieve symptoms may be difficult.[55]

- Legislative processes continue to be used to promote or challenge aspects of the law that permits AD in , for example, Canada where the Quebec Government is considering making severe disability an eligibility criterion to access AD.[56] Challenges are being entered[57] in courts to attempt to move the eligibility for MAiD in Canada back to the 2020 status where death had to be "reasonably foreseeable" for a patient to be eligible.

- We discussed the challenges and delays surrounding including mental illness in the eligibility of MAiD in Canada in Chapter 2. Some disabled people and advocates see this proposal as flawed and are deeply concerned that gaps in mental healthcare provision could lead to its inappropriate use or abuse.[58] In the Netherlands where mental health is included in the eligibility criteria for AD, the proportion of AD cases for which the unbearable suffering is non-somatic illness is low. There are, however, concerns about this and ongoing debate.[59]

- Individual experiences and views continue to be a feature of the literature in disadvantage, disability and AD (for example, Refs.[60–65]) stimulating thought and further discussions of these complex issues.

The disability organisations and movement have a long-standing commitment to autonomy for disabled people who must take their own decisions. They are concerned that disabled people, along with poor people and other disadvantaged groups, might be pressurised into ending their lives without proper consideration or even against their will. The mid-20th century experiences of so called "mercy killing" are not consigned to history and healthcare professionals at that time did not prevent those despicable excesses. Some have expressed the view that some of the debates about AD have lacked respect for the views of disabled and disadvantaged people. Even when laws are framed around the eligibility of Terminal illness, they may fear that there is a "slippery slope" towards wider eligibility criteria to include unbearable suffering from long term illness without a defined limitation of life expectation. From that change they may feel it is a shorter step to disability alone being considered as a criterion for AD. Could that lead to coercion being applied for disabled people to end their lives?

There is no robust evidence that in jurisdictions which permit AD, either for terminal illness or for unbearable suffering, that disabled or disadvantaged people are inappropriately overrepresented people in the statistics for the numbers of people that access AD. That is reassuring but probably not yet entirely convincing given the dynamic nature of changes in legislation and the incomplete data collection in the earlier studies of more mature AD systems. Disabled and disadvantaged people will be as vulnerable to the major fatal illnesses, most commonly cancer, which lead people to access AD in permissive jurisdictions. Their access to all end-of-life care with all its choices must be provided and delivered in a sensitive, professional and empathic way.

Twycross[66] takes an overview of many of these issues and, while accepting that AD is likely to become legal in the UK in the next few years, remains concerned that the benefits that are anticipated for the small number(likely 1–2%) of patients who access AD at the end of their lives, must not be outweighed by the reduction in access to high quality Palliative Care or by the creation of disincentives to people to seek and benefit from such care. While many patients may be reassured to know that they have a range of choices at the end of their lives, and a few may choose AD, we have to develop laws, care services and processes which protect all patients from inadequate or inappropriate care. Twycross suggests that could be best attained by having AD services separated from the mainstreams of healthcare and accessed by referral.[66] Such arguments may find favour with some healthcare professions and disciplines, not least because there is good data showing that members of most medical disciplines have a smaller proportion of people who support AD than the general public in the UK.

The team which has brought together this book and its predecessor, have held to the view that the decision to permit AD belongs to the public and their legislators in Parliament. It is the job of well-informed professionals is to advise and devise safe and effective ways of ensuring that the benefits of AD for those who freely choose it at the end of their lives are delivered safely and effectively and without disadvantaging others. There are very important points that everyone involved will need to take from the international and national opinions and commentary on the issues discussed in this Chapter.

Cultural, especially religious, beliefs and sensitivities are a central issue on these decisions and planning. While a majority of people in the UK and the jurisdictions which permit AD seem to be supportive of AD for terminal illness, there are in all these countries and jurisdictions a substantial minority of people whose beliefs are profoundly opposed the AD especially on religious grounds. These views are long lasting and unlikely to become less prominent in the foreseeable future. They have to be respected in the operation of AD systems and procedure but, for example, always allowing appropriate conscience-driven decisions for staff and patients.

The views of disabled people on AD are divided. Some seeing AD as a real threat with the fear that their lives may be less valued and they could be inappropriately pressurised into accessed AD. Other see AD as offering them autonomy and self-determination in they were to find themselves facing a terminal illness. Appropriate laws and regulations may address some of these fears and the international experience and data does not show an excess of disabled people among those taking up access to AD. However, the long-term data are not generally as detailed as we would wish, and further meticulous monitoring is needed. Disabled people must be involved in the oversight and monitoring processes of any new systems for AD in any jurisdictions.

References

1. Bloomer MJ, Saffer L, Hewitt J, et al. Maybe for unbearable suffering: diverse racial, ethnic and cultural perspectives of assisted dying. A scoping review. Palliat. Med. 2024;38(9):968–980.

2. Braun KL. Do Hawaii residents support physician-assisted death? A comparison of five ethnic groups. Hawaii Med J. 1998;57:529–534.

3. Braun KL, Nichols R. Cultural issues in death and dying. Hawaii Med J. 1996;55:260–264.

4. Braun KL, Tanji VM, Heck R. Support for physician-assisted suicide: exploring the impact of ethnicity and attitudes toward planning for death. Gerontologist. 2001;41:51–60.

5. Cain CL, McCleskey S. Expanded definitions of the 'good death'? Race, ethnicity and medical aid in dying. Social Health Illness. 2019;41:1175–1191.

6. Caralis PV, Davis B, Wright K, et al. The influence of ethnicity and race on attitudes toward advance directives, life-prolonging treatments, and euthanasia. J Clin Eth. 1993;4:155–165.

7. Espino DV, Macias RL, Wood RC, et al. Physician-assisted suicide attitudes of older Mexican American and non-Hispanic White adults: does ethnicity make a difference? J Am Geriatric Soc. 2010;58:1370–1375.

8. Lichtenstein RL, Alcser KH, Corning AD, et al. Black/white differences in attitudes toward physician-assisted suicide. J National Med Assoc 1997;89:125–133.

9. Mouton CP, Espino DV, Esparza Y, et al. Attitudes toward assisted suicide among community-dwelling Mexican Americans. Clin Gerontol. 2001;22:81–92.

10. Periyakoil VS, Kraemer H, Neri E. Multi-ethnic attitudes toward physician-assisted death in California and Hawaii. J Palliat Med. 2016;19:1060–1065.

11. Wasserman J, Clair JM, Ritchey FJ. Racial differences in attitudes toward euthanasia. Omega. 2005;52:263–287.

12. Ahaddour C, Van den Branden S, Broeckaert B. "God is the giver and taker of life": Muslim beliefs and attitudes regarding assisted suicide and euthanasia. AJOB Empir Bioeth. 2018;9:1–11.

13. Baeke G, Wils J-P, Broeckaert B. 'We are (not) the master of our body': elderly Jewish women's attitudes towards euthanasia and assisted suicide. Eth Health. 2011;16:259–278.

14. Baeke G, Wils J-P, Broeckaert B. "It's in God's Hands": the attitudes of elderly Muslim women in Antwerp, Belgium, toward active termination of life. AJOB Prim Res. 2012;3:36–47.

15. Waddell C, McNamara B. The stereotypical fallacy: comparison of Anglo and Chinese Australians' thoughts about facing death. Mortality. 1997;2:149–161.

16. Stolz E, Mayerl H, Gasser-Steiner P, et al. Attitudes towards assisted suicide and euthanasia among care-dependent older adults (50+) in Austria: the role of socio-demographics, religiosity, physical illness, psychological distress, and social isolation. BMC Med Eth. 2017;18:1–13.

17. Dorji N, Lapierre S, Dransart DAC. Perception of medical assistance in dying among Asian Buddhists living in Montreal, Canada. Omega. 2022;85:579–603.

18. Jylhänkangas L, Smets T, Cohen J, et al. Descriptions of euthanasia as social representations: comparing the views of Finnish physicians and religious professionals. Social Health Illness. 2014;36:354–368.

19. https://www.opinium.com

20. Opinium 2024. Will public opinion translate into legislative change? https://www.opinium.com/resource-center/will-public-opinion-translate-into-legislative-change which includes a link to the Excel Spreadsheet.

21. Kozlov E, Luth EA, Nemeth S, et al. Knowledge of and preferences for medical aid in dying. JAMA Netw Open. 2025;8(2):e2461495.

22. Dehkhoda A, Frey R, Carey M, et al. Health professionals' understanding and attitude towards the End of Life Choice Act 2019: a secondary analysis of Manatū Hauora– Ministry of Health workforce surveys. N Z Med J. 2023;136(1576):11–31.

23. Grundnig JS, Roehe MA, Trost C, et al. Attitudes of undergraduate medical students towards end-of-life decisions: a systematic review of influencing factors. BMC Med Educ. 2025;25(1):642.

24. Hawrelak E, Harper L, Reddon JR, et al. Canadian undergraduates' perspectives on medical assistance in dying (MAiD): a quantitative study. J Palliat Care. 2022;37(3):352–358.

25. Mahnoor; Shahid AN, Shafiq H, et al. Attitude of undergraduate medical students towards euthanasia and physician-assisted suicide: a cross-sectional study. J Pak Med Assoc. 2024;74(5):1022–1025.

26. Hamer MK, Baugh CM, Bolcic-Jankovic D, et al. Conscience-based barriers to medical aid in dying: a survey of colorado physicians. J Gen Intern Med. 2024;39(16):3138–3145.

27. Wiebe E, Sum B, Kelly M, et al. Forced and chosen transfers for medical assistance in dying (MAiD) before and during the COVID 19 pandemic: a mixed methods study. Death Stud. 2022;46(9):2266–2272.

28. Takimoto Y, Nabeshima T. Disparity in attitudes regarding assisted dying among physicians and the general public in Japan. BMC Med Ethics. 2025;26(1):7.

29. Borovecki A, Curkovic M, Nikodem K, et al. Attitudes about withholding or withdrawing life-prolonging treatment, euthanasia, assisted suicide, and physician assisted suicide: a cross-sectional survey among the general public in Croatia. BMC Med Ethics. 2022;23(1):13.

30. Bachmetjev B, Airapetian A, Zablockis R. Attitude of the Lithuanian public toward medical assistance in dying: a cross-sectional study. Healthcare (Basel). 2024;12(6):626.

31. Wajid M, Rajkumar E, Romate J. What enhances the quality of death and dying? A perspective from patients with terminal cancer. Int J Palliat Nurs. 2024;30(9):496–508.

32. Parra Jounou I, Triviño-Caballero R, Cruz-Piqueras M. For, against, and beyond: healthcare professionals' positions on medical assistance in dying in Spain. BMC Med Eth. 2024;25(1):69.

33. Assisted Dying. Disability Rights UK opposes the Terminally Ill Adults (End of Life) Bill. https://www.disabilityrightsuk.org/assisted-dying?srsltid=AfmBOoqlsPW-ckj3cTdEXZ62jK4B0u3-WSUtd7IrCe1XqvkbCQACqyPG

34. Disability Rights UK's Position on Assisted Dying. https://www.disabilityrightsuk.org/news/disability-rights-uk%E2%80%99s-position-assisted-dying

35. Disability rights campaigners urge MPs and peers to back assisted dying bill. https://www.theguardian.com/society/2024/oct/24/disability-rights-campaigners-urge-mps-peers-back-assisted-dying-bill

36. Disabled people's organisations unite to oppose assisted suicide bill that has 'far-reaching implications'. https://www.disabilitynewsservice.com/disabled-peoples-organisations-unite-to-oppose-assisted-suicide-bill-that-has-far-reaching-implications

37. My Death, My Decision. The views of disabled people within the assisted dying debate. https://www.mydeath-mydecision.org.uk/2024/05/13/the-views-of-disabled-people-within-the-assisted-dying-debate/

38. Devastation as Assisted Dying Bill Passes. https://www.disabilityrightsuk.org/news/devastation-assisted-dying-bill-passes

39. Box G, Chambaere K. Views of disability rights organisations on assisted dying legislation in England, Wales and Scotland: an analysis of position statements. J Med Eth. 2021;47(12):e64.

40. Lewis P. How do permissive regimes regulate assisted dying? In: Board R, Bennett MI, Lewis P, Wagstaff J, Selby P, eds. End-of-life choices for cancer patients. An international perspective. Oxford: EBN Health, 2020.

41. Battin MP, Vander Heide A, Ganzini L, et al. Legal physician-assisted dying in Oregon and the Netherlands: evidence concerning the impact on patients in vulnerable groups. J Med Eth. 2007;33:591–597.

42. Rietjens JAC, Deschepper R, Pasman R, et al. Medical end-of-life decisions: does its use differ in vulnerable patient groups? A systematic review and meta- analysis. Social Sci Med. 2012;74:1282–1287.

43. Steck M, Egger M, Maessen T, et al. Euthanasia and assisted suicide in selected European countries and US states: systematic literature review. Med Care. 2013;51:938–944.19E.

44. Emanuel J, Onwuteaka-Philipsen BD, Urwin JW, et al. Attitudes and practices of euthanasia and physician-assisted suicide in the United States, Canada, and Europe. J Am Med Assoc. 2016;316:79–90.

45. Dierickx S, Deliens L, Cohen J, et al. Comparison of the expression and granting of requests for euthanasia in Belgium in 2007 v 2013. JAMA Intern Med. 2015;175:1703–1706.

46. Colburn B. Disability-based arguments against assisted dying laws. Bioethics. 2022;36(6):680–686.

47. Redelmeier DA, Ng K., Thiruchelvam D, et al. Association of socioeconomic status with medical assistance in dying: a case–control analysis. BMJ Open. 2021;11(5):1–10.

48. Tran M, Honarmand K, Sibbald R, et al. Socioeconomic status and medical assistance in dying: a regional descriptive study. J Palliat Care. 2022;37(3):359–365.

49. Asada Y, Campbell LA, Grignon M, et al. Importance of investigating vulnerabilities in health and social service provision among requestors of medical assistance in dying. Lancet Reg Health Am. 2024;35:100810.

50. Bérubé A, Tapp D, Dupéré S, et al. Do socioeconomic factors influence knowledge, attitudes, and representations of end-of-life practices? A cross-sectional study. J Palliat Care. 2025;40(2):152–161.

51. Anderson JB, Cacciapuoti M, Day H, et al. The impact of legalizing medical aid in dying on patient trust: a randomized controlled survey Study. J Palliat Med. 2024;27(11):1459–1466.

52. Pope TM, Shavelson L, Battin MP, et al. Permit assisted self-administration: a response to open peer commentaries on neurologic diseases and medical aid in dying: aid-in-dying laws create an underclass of patients based on disability. Am J Bioeth. 2023;23(9):W9–W14.

53. Wright MS. Current medical aid-in-dying laws discriminate against individuals with disabilities. Am J Bioeth. 2023;23(9):33–35.

54. Shavelson L, Pope TM, Battin MP, et al. Neurologic diseases and medical aid in dying: aid-in-dying laws create an underclass of patients based on disability. Am J Bioeth. 2023;23(9):5–15.

55. Hopkins SA, Price A, Etkind SN. Why we need to consider frailty in the assisted dying debate. Age Ageing. 2025;54(2):afaf028.

56. Dyer O. Assisted dying: Quebec extends eligibility to cover severe disability and allow procedure in outdoor spaces. BMJ. 2023;381:1361.

57. Dyer O. Assisted dying: disability advocates launch legal challenge to Canada's law. BMJ. 2024;387:q2161.

58. Chown S. Disability community feels ignored in Canada's assisted dying expansion. BMJ. 2024;385:q806.

59. Tuffrey-Wijne I, Curfs L, Hollins S, et al. Euthanasia and physician-assisted suicide in people with intellectual disabilities and/or autism spectrum disorders: investigation of 39 Dutch case reports (2012-2021). BJPsych Open. 2023;9(3):e87.

60. Coelho R, Maher J, Gaind KS, et al. The realities of medical assistance in dying in Canada. Palliat Support Care. 2023;21(5):871–878.

61. Hughes T. Assisted dying poses significant risks to disabled people. BMJ. 2024;387:q2730.

62. Downar J, MacDonald S, Buchman SJ. Medical assistance in dying, palliative care, safety, and structural vulnerability. Palliat Med. 2023;26(9):1175–1179.

63. Gallagher R, Coelho R, Violette PD, et al. Response to medical assistance in dying, palliative care, safety, and structural vulnerability. J Palliat Med. 2023;26(12):1610–1617.

64. Atkins CGK. A disabled bioethicist's critique of Canada's medical assistance in dying (MAID). Am J Bioeth. 2023;23(11):102–104.

65. Memorandum by Dr Tom Shakespeare. https://publications.parliament.uk/pa/ld200405/ldselect/ldasdy/86/4120223.htm

66. Twycross R. Assisted dying: principles, possibilities, and practicalities. An English physician's perspective. BMC Palliat Care. 2024;23(1):99.

Chapter 9: What Do We Know About the Patients' and Caregivers' Experience?

The literature on the experience of patients, their caregivers, families and friends when someone chooses an assisted death, is relatively modest compared to the literature describing experiences of professionals involved in the delivery of the service. However, a number of studies look at this important area in detail from both the perspective of the patient themselves and also the families and caregivers involved in the process. This is an important resource which can help inform how to develop an AD service to appropriately reflect the needs of all involved.

Martin et al. conducted a scoping review of 19 articles from a number of countries on the topic "Qualities of the dying experience of persons who access medical assistance in dying".[1] They concluded *"Our review indicates that allowing Medical Assistance in Dying (MAiD) access offers an element of control in a dying situation for the individuals and families that may not be possible within the context of a natural death, since the person is typically awake and able to engage with care partners at the time of death".*[1] The literature describes positive aspects of AD: how individuals can set out their own time scale for their death, determine who will be present, experience less physical pain and suffering, have an increased sense of autonomy and dignity. Family members can visit, say their goodbyes and complete any unfinished conversations or business. They point to the importance of MAiD providers ensuring careful planning taking into account the wishes and needs of patients and families to ensure ongoing open communication.

Buchbinder et al. conducted in-depth interviews of lay caregivers in Vermont, USA who were mostly close friends of the patient choosing AD and who supported them on the day of death.[2] Vermont introduced the Patient Choice and Control at the End-of-Life Act in 2013. Buchbinder's findings[2] support the conclusions of Martin et al.[1] and emphasise the tremendous support given by family and close friends and the deep implications, both moral and social, of the involvement in the process.

The role of relatives during the period of time when the patient is considering a request for AD was studied in the Netherlands by Snijdewind et al.[3] and Dees et al.[4] Relatives have an important and influential role in the decision-taking process and the management of its complexities which may be follow the expected course but can be readily disrupted by personal and logistic factors or when, for example, the illness does not follow the expected course.

Assisted Dying (MAiD) became legal in Canada in 2016 and at the 5-year point in its implementation, Goldberg et al.,[5] in their review of the literature, acknowledged that, while family caregivers are the backbone of the care provided, there was still little knowledge of the impact on them in Canada and globally and the literature can be difficult to interpret with confidence because methodologies are variable.[5] While most family members support the decision of their loved ones to seek AD, there are discrepancies between the discussions reported by the patients and family members.[5] Family members viewed the experience for their loved ones of AD as being likely to be better than the death they expected from natural causes. An earlier systematic review by Hendry et al.[6] also concluded the bereaved caregivers viewed MAiD as making a positive contribution and preserving dignity, alleviating suffering and respecting what the patient had wanted.[6] Smith et al.[7] in Oregon compared scores in a Quality of Dying structured questionnaire between bereaved care givers of patients who had experienced AD compared to a natural death.

The quality of death was rated more highly by those whose relatives had experienced AD.[7] Laparle et al. confirmed the finding that there was no difference in the grief experience of individuals who lost loved ones through AD or a natural death.[8] This is further supported by a review of the literature on bereavement and grief following AD by Srinivasan.[9] Following 22 interviews of bereaved family members in Oregon there was no evidence that family members grieving for a loved one's assisted or non-assisted death experienced different degrees of prolonged grieving or depression and those who were grieving following an assisted death reported that they had been more prepared.[9] However, some bereaved family members reported feeling of "self-blame" following an assisted death and in other studies, a small number of relatives who encounter moral dilemmas with the MAiD decision experience concern throughout the MAiD process and beyond shown by Gamondi et al.[10]

Serota et al.[11] have studied the impact of AD on families and caregivers in Canada using narrative interviews. They have explored and described family discordance, internal conflict, concerns about the legal position, logistic challenges and managing disclosure, as factors which can have an impact on bereavement after AD[12] and constructed narratives which convey the vision which is sought and expected for MAiD (a Dignified Narrative) with two others (a Traumatic Narrative and an Unjust Narrative) which will stimulate consideration of the complexity of the challenge of delivering AD to the standard sought by patients and health professionals.[12]

Studies of the mental health of families and caregivers after a patient accessed AD are not common but are broadly reassuring that there appears to be little difference in outcome between caregivers and families of those who died naturally and those who had assisted deaths.[13] Those whose loved ones accessed AD might have had less complicated grief.[14] There is consistent support in the literature for the case to enhance not only the support for patients who are in an AD pathway but also for their families and caregivers before, during and after the assisted death.[15,16] Renckens et al.[17] studied aftercare meetings with families after AD of a relative and found provision to be patchy and suggested that follow up support may be valuable in improving mental health and well-being. An important point for AD providers and policymakers to consider.

Feigin et al.[18] in a notable and uncommon study, interviewed three bereaved family members who had assisted their loved ones in dying before the legalisation of the procedures in New Zealand, resulting in criminal proceedings, imprisonment, home detention or discharge. They all experienced immense stress and turmoil but felt that their concern to "do the right thing" overrode concerns about consequences.[18] In Switzerland, in the absence of evidence of self-interest, it is not illegal to assist someone to die including the provision of medication for self-administration. Both foreign visitors and Swiss nationals have therefore been able to access AD since 1937 and there has been a substantial increase in AD over recent decades. This is somewhat controversial, and guidelines are issued by Swiss Academy of Medical Sciences.[19] Despite this lengthy experience of AD in Switzerland, there may still be dilemmas facing the families of patients who seek AD, and feelings of isolation, culpability and social stigma are reported.[20,21]

Al Rabadi et al. summarised the Oregon and Washington State data on Assisted Dying.[22] Oregon introduced the Death with Dignity Act in 1994 and implemented it in 1997; Washington State introduced Assisted Dying in 2008. The most common reasons given for pursuing AD were loss of autonomy (87%), impaired quality of life (86%) and loss of dignity (69%). These reasons are in keeping with the literature in general and it seems that the symptom burden in patients requesting AD is similar to that of patients who do not request it.[23] In the Oregon data 96% reported AD with no complication, but complication rates were reported in 4% of cases, most commonly due to difficulty swallowing or vomiting the oral medications required. The median time to coma after drug ingestion was 5 min and median time to death was 25 min. However, the total ranges of times reported for onset of coma was 1–660 min and for death was 1–6240 min. Eight patients woke up after drug ingestion and a period of coma.[22] It is likely that the prolonged periods to coma or death in some patients are traumatic for patients and families. Carers' grief can last longer when the experience is not successful in facilitating a perceived "good death"[9] and a smooth and peaceful procedure is of upmost importance.

The crucial role of a family centred approach to AD is highlighted by Nissim et al.[23] in Toronto. They interviewed 18 family caregivers at least 6 months after the loved one's death through AD focussing on the day of death and the experience of the family.[23] Caregivers were grateful and positive but described the day as "potentially jarring and unsettling". Factors which were mentioned as having potential to unsettle were: attuned support from the clinical team, preparation of clinical details, congruence between the setting and the importance of the event, active participation and ceremony and the pace of the procedure.

To gain further insight Canadian and Australian researchers have collaborated to explore how to improve the experience of AD by listening to the feedback from families and caregivers[24] Interviews with 67 caregivers suggested 6 themes for improvement: improved content and dissemination of information about AD; proactive development of policies and procedures; address institutional objections from the top down; develop grief resources and peer support; amend laws to address legal barriers; engage with and act on feedback from families and caregivers.[24] Lewis et al.[25] in three Australian States explored the "choreography of a good death" in interviews with 42 caregivers bringing out the complexity of the wish to fulfil the patient's wishes against a background of institutional and cultural complexities and tensions. Young et al.[26] in New Zealand sought to establish methods to find the optimal timing for AD in the patients' journey whereby choosing a date to die should be in accordance with patients wishes but cannot be untangled from the practical aspects of AD such as the providers availability and timeframes outlined in law. White et al.,[27] in Queensland in a recent extraordinary collaboration between healthcare professionals, lawyers and creative writers, interviewed 32 caregivers and a patient whose responses expressed gratitude for the experience in five poems. There is an emerging literature on the impact of cultural diversity and place-based care issues on the processes and caregiver and family outcomes of AD,[28,29] which we discussed in more detail in Chapter 1. It is clear that much more work and research need to be done in this area to ensure those accessing AD have their beliefs and cultures respected and appropriate provisions are made.

Martin et al.[1] concluded "In summary, it appears a good death is one that exists beyond the single moment of death and extends a wider influence, thereby shaping the experiences of those that shared the journey leading up to the assisted death. Our scoping review discusses several attributes of good death among people accessing MAiD, including increased symptom control and reduced suffering, respecting individual autonomy, dignified dying, increased sense of connectedness, transcendence, and peaceful death. Our findings support that MAiD could increase the likelihood of experiencing a good death. Our review also informs the providers that MAiD access should allow careful planning as per the needs and wishes of the patients and their families alongside open and ongoing communication. The MAiD journey is one in which emotional connection can strengthen between individual, family members, and their clinical care providers."

The data around patient and carer givers experience of AD is generally positive and provides reassurance that AD can provide a 'good death'. Patients who opt for AD and those who opt for a natural death and receive palliative care, have similar symptom burdens,[30] which reinforces the absolute need that all of the options available to patients at the end of their lives are readily accessible and of high quality.

It is crucial that we continue to monitor and learn from the experiences of those accessing AD and those who do not. This includes making appropriate information, communication and support available to patients and caregivers at all stages of the process: before, during and after, and in the context of their culture, beliefs and background. This approach should ensure safe and effective services for those that choose AD and those who do not.

References

1. Martin T, Freeman S, Lalani N, et al. Qualities of the dying experience of persons who access medical assistance in dying: a scoping review. Death Stud. 2023;47(9):1033–1043.

2. Buchbinder M, Ojo E, Knio L, et al. Caregivers' experiences with medical aid-in-dying in Vermont: a qualitative study. J Pain Symp. Manag. 2018,56(6):936–943.

3. Snijdewind MC, van Tol DG, Onwuteaka-Philipsen BD, et al. Complexities in euthanasia or physician-assisted suicide as perceived by Dutch physicians and patients' relatives. J Pain Sympt Manag 2014;48(6):1125–1134.

4. Dees MK, Vernooij-Dassen MJ, Dekkers WJ, et al. Perspectives of decision-making in requests for euthanasia: qualitative research among patients, relatives and treating physicians in the Netherlands. Palliat Med. 2012;27(1):27–37.

5. Goldberg R, Nissim R, An E, et al. Impact of medical assistance in dying (MAiD) on family caregivers. BMJ Support Palliat Care. 2021;11(1):107–114.

6. Hendry M, Pasterfield D, Lewis R, et al. Why do we want the right to die? A systematic review of the international literature on the views of patients, carers and the public on assisted dying. Palliat Med. 2013;27(1):13–26.

7. Smith KA, Goy ER, Harvath TA, et al. Quality of death and dying in patients who request physician-assisted death. J Palliat Med. 2011;14(4):445–450.

8. Laperle P, Achille M, Ummel D. To lose a loved one by medical assistance in dying or by natural death with palliative care: a mixed methods comparison of grief experiences. Omega (Westport). 2024;89(3):931–953.

9. Srinivasan EG. Bereavement and the Oregon Death with Dignity Act: how does assisted death impact grief? Death Stud. 2019;43(10):647–655.

10. Gamondi C, Pott M, Forbes K, et al. Exploring the experiences of bereaved families involved in assisted suicide in Southern Switzerland: a qualitative study. BMJ Support Palliat Care. 2015;5(2):146–152.

11. Serota K, Buchman DZ, Atkinson M. Mapping MAiD discordance: a qualitative analysis of the factors complicating MAiD bereavement in Canada. Qual Health Res. 2024;34(3):195–204.

12. Serota K, Atkinson M, Upshur R, et al. Dignity Narratives in Complex MAiD Bereavement Stories: A Critical Qualitative Analysis. Narrative Inquiry in Bioethics. 2025;15(3):1–17. Johns Hopkins University Press, 2025.

13. Ganzini L, Goy ER, Dobscha SK, et al. Mental health outcomes of family members of Oregonians who request physician aid in dying. J Pain Symptom Manage. 2009;38(6):807–815.

14. Swarte NB, van der Lee ML, van der Bom JG, et al. Effects of euthanasia on the bereaved family and friends: a cross sectional study. BMJ. 2003;327(7408):189.

15. Oczkowski SJW, Crawshaw DE, Austin P, et al. How can we improve the experiences of patients and families who request medical assistance in dying? A multi-centre qualitative study. BMC Palliat Care. 2021;20(1):185.

16. Vissers S, Gilissen J, Cohen J, et al. The support needs of patients requesting medical aid in dying and their relatives: a qualitative study using semi-structured interviews and written narratives. Int J Public Health. 2024;69:1–10.

17. Renckens SC, Pasman HR, van der Heide A, et al. Aftercare provision for bereaved relatives following euthanasia or physician-assisted suicide: a cross-sectional questionnaire study among physicians. Int J Public Health. 2024;69:1607346.

18. Feigin S, Owens RG, Goodyear-Smith F. Helping a loved one die: the act of assisted dying in New Zealand. Mortality. 2019;24(1):95–110.

19. https://www.alliancevita.org/en/2023/10/assisted-suicide-in-switzerland/

20. Gaignard ME, Hurst S. A qualitative study on existential suffering and assisted suicide in Switzerland. BMC Med Ethics. 2019;20(1):34.

21. Gamondi C, Pott M, Payne S. Families' experiences with patients who died after assisted suicide: a retrospective interview study in southern Switzerland. Ann Oncol. 2013;24:1639–1644.

22. Al Rabadi L, LeBlanc M, Bucy T, et al. Trends in medical aid in dying in Oregon and Washington. JAMA Netw Open. 2019;2(8):e198648.

23. Nissim R, Chu P, Stere A, et al. "Walk me through the final day": a thematic analysis study on the family caregiver experience of the Medical Assistance in Dying procedure day. Palliat Med. 2024;38(6):660–668.

24. Jeanneret R, Close E, Willmott L, et al. Patients' and caregivers' suggestions for improving assisted dying regulation: a qualitative study in Australia and Canada. Health Expect. 2024;27(3):e14107.

25. Lewis S, La Brooy C, Kerridge I, et al. Choreographing a good death: carers' experiences and practices of enacting assisted dying. Sociol Health Illn. 2024;46(7):1345–1363.

26. Young JE, Lyons AC, Dew K, et al. Is there a right time to die? How patients, families and assisted dying providers decide on and anticipate a date with death. Death Stud. 2024;12:1–13.

27. White BP, Jeanneret R, Holland-Batt S, et al. 'This is perfect, thank you': research poetry on gratitude for voluntary assisted dying in Victoria, Australia. Australas J Ageing. 2025;44(2):e70019.

28. Bloomer MJ, Saffer L, Hewitt J, et al. Maybe for unbearable suffering: diverse racial, ethnic and cultural perspectives of assisted dying. A scoping review. Palliat Med. 2024;38(9):968–980.

29. Sedgwick M, Brassolotto J, Manduca-Barone A. Rural healthcare professionals' participation in Medical Assistance in Dying (MAiD): beyond a binary decision. BMC Palliat Care. 2024;23(1):107.

30. Russell KB, Forbes C, Qi S, et al. End-of-life symptom burden among patients with cancer who were provided Medical Assistance in Dying (MAID): a longitudinal propensity-score-matched cohort study. Cancers (Basel). 2024;16(7):1294.

Chapter 10: Medical Jurisprudence

Introduction

It is well recognised that laws affect and modulate health in multiple ways.[1] One impactful interaction between law and health is through various social determinants of health, such as nutrition, housing and environment, which are shaped and reinforced by legal frameworks. Another impact arises from laws that govern healthcare systems and care options that are available to people. In this broader context, assisted dying – as a final extension of healthcare - becomes an important legal consideration.

Understanding that health has critical legal determinants includes recognising that medicine is essentially a social enterprise. Consequently, it can be argued that medical ethics and professional obligations are fundamentally governed by the law, rather than the converse.[2] Within this framework, assisted dying is not entirely or exclusively a medical issue; it is also a major legal concern.[3]

The present chapter explores the statutory provisions of the *Terminally Ill Adults (End of Life) Bill*[4] (hereinafter the 'Bill') within the underpinning legal philosophy - or jurisprudence - that informs medical practice in the UK. Jurisprudence addresses the nature of law, its connection with morality (the distinction between right and wrong), and its function in society. A study of jurisprudence often revolves around questions of what we mean by justice or fairness, and whether and how the law reflects the underlying conception of justice. Thus, jurisprudence alerts us to problems of fairness that might pervade existing law, and it helps us to navigate these gaps responsibly.

Understanding jurisprudence requires some familiarity with the UK's common law tradition. In a common law system, legal principles are developed through judicial decisions rather than solely by parliamentary legislation. When a legal dispute arises, judges interpret and apply both relevant statutes as well as prior judicial rulings in similar cases, thereby building a body of case law or legal doctrine. The common law evolves over time, allowing for flexibility and adaptation.

In contrast, many jurisdictions outside the UK follow a civil law system, in which legal rules are codified in comprehensive statutes and legal codes, and judges play a more limited role in shaping the law. Judicial decisions in civil law countries do not generally have binding precedent; instead, the primary function of judges is to apply the written code to individual cases. Legal development occurs principally through legislative reform rather than judicial interpretation.

Common law systems are found in countries with historical ties to the British Empire, including the United States, Canada, Australia, India, and New Zealand. Civil law systems, derived from Roman law and the Napoleonic Code, are used in most of continental Europe (e.g. France, Germany, Italy), Latin America, parts of Asia (e.g. Japan, South Korea), and much of Africa. Some jurisdictions, such as South Africa and Scotland, incorporate elements of both systems and are considered mixed or hybrid legal systems.

In both common law and civil law, jurisprudential analysis is important for grasping how current medical practices align with existing medical law as well as societal expectations. A sound understanding of jurisprudence can thus equip doctors to adopt a legally and ethically approach to the Bill, assuming that it is enacted. The focus of the present chapter is limited to analysis of UK law in the context of assisted dying. However, the broad principles that emerge from the jurisprudential analysis in this chapter are likely to apply internationally and should serve to address global legal concerns around assisted dying.

In the discussion that follows, section I introduces the common law principle of public interest that exempts doctors who provide assistance in dying from criminal charges. Section II explains that individual determination overrides public interest in cases of declining treatment or withdrawing life-supporting treatment. However, a particular understanding of liberty that was advanced by Isaiah Berlin, a political philosopher (section III), helps us to understand why public interest is prioritised over individual self-determination for requesting or demanding certain treatments (section IV). It is for this reason that parliamentary legislation is necessary to establish that assisted dying is in the public interest; simply self-determination does not suffice. Section V deals with the question of whether assisted dying is a medical treatment. Section VI explains the legal principles of shared decision-making that would apply if assisted dying is regarded as a medical treatment. Sections VII and VIII then point out ethical dilemmas in decision-making that can arise both for doctors who choose to participate in assisted dying and for those who choose not to do so, respectively. Section IX concludes this chapter.

The medical exception to the criminal law

A central legal concern regarding assisted dying is that doctors who facilitate it could be prosecuted for manslaughter or even murder under current law. The Bill addresses this concern directly: assuming that it becomes law, it ensures that doctors who assist in dying in accordance with the Bill's provisions will not be criminally or civilly liable. The Bill explicitly affirms these exemptions from criminal and civil law.

This legal exemption mirrors the approach that the law already takes towards various medical interventions that might otherwise constitute criminal acts. Consider, for example, a surgical operation. Why is the surgeon not subject to a criminal charge, when the infliction of a wound by one person on another, in any other circumstance, would be an assault? It is because there is a well-established line of jurisprudence that 'proper medical treatment' is in the 'public interest'[5]; and, so, it is not a criminal act.[6] Accordingly, surgical acts done with consent and for therapeutic purposes are legally justified.

By extension, if the Bill is enacted, it could be inferred that Parliament has deemed assisted dying to be in the public interest, interpreted broadly as the common interest of the British public. Therefore, public interest provides a justification for exempting medical assistance of dying from the scope of criminal law.

Prioritisation of self-determination over public interest for refusing and withdrawing medical treatment

The reliance on public reason for exempting proper medical treatment from the criminal law is intriguing and bi-pronged. On one hand, the law affirms that a competent patient has the right to refuse treatment – even if the decision is unwise or leads to death. As established by the House of Lords:

> 'A doctor has no right to proceed in the face of objection, even if it is plain to all, including the patient, that adverse consequences and even death will or may ensue' (pg. 891H).[5]

At the same times, courts have acknowledged that refusals of treatment can create substantial tension because there is a 'very strong public interest in preserving the life and health of all citizens' (pg. 115G).[7] Consequently, as explained by the Court of Appeal, a patient's refusal of treatment:

> [G]ives rise to a conflict between two interests, that of the patient and that of the society in which he lives. The patient's interest consists of his right to self-determination – his right to live his own life how he wishes, even if it will damage his health or lead to his premature death. Society's interest is in upholding the concept that all human life if sacred and that it should be preserved if at all possible (pg. 112E).[7]

Nonetheless, senior courts have been consistent in holding that each person's right to self-determination takes precedence over the public interest in preserving life in cases involving the refusal of medical treatment. This prioritisation of self-determination for refusing treatment extends to withdrawing life-supporting treatment and allowing a person to die.[5,8] These legal principles applies equally for both people with decision-making capacity as well as best interest decision-making by others for people without capacity.

This prioritisation of self-determination over the public interest does not, however, extend to cases in which a patient demands or requests a specific treatment. Here, the law draws a sharp distinction between refusing treatment and requesting it: a crucial distinction for understanding the legal controversy surrounding assisted dying. Whilst treatment refusal/withdrawal and consequent death are well accepted, the legal right to access assisted dying has not traditionally existed.

A cogent explanation for the distinction between treatment-refusals and treatment-demands is supplied a particular conceptualisation of liberty that was put forward by Isaiah Berlin, a well-known, 20th century political philosopher. Liberty or freedom serves as a forerunner of the principles of self-determination and autonomy that are prized in modern medical practice. As recently discussed elsewhere, Berlin's ideas on liberty are especially relevant to the debate on assisted dying.[9] The next section deals with Berlin's ideas of liberty, and the succeeding section then discusses the common law on requests for treatment, as might pertain to assisted dying, within this framework of liberty.

Two senses of liberty

Berlin articulated two core senses of (or ideas within) liberty: negative and positive.[10] Negative liberty refers to an individual's 'freedom from' external interference: a protected, personal space in which a person may act without unjustified intrusion by others, including the state. This does not imply the absence of any regulation, but rather that a just society must clearly demarcate which types of interference are unacceptable from those that are tied to the privilege of living in that society.

These restrictions - the scope of negative liberty - vary across societies, according to the underlying political philosophy to which each society subscribes.[11] For instance, John Stuart Mill argued that we are free to do:

> [A]s we like, subject to such consequences as may follow: without impediment from our fellow-creatures, so long as what we do does not harm them, even though they should think our conduct foolish, perverse or wrong (pg. 15).[12]

Thus, Millian liberty holds that restrictive influences or restraints can be justified only by the 'harm' principle; people are free to do whatever they choose, provided that they do not harm others. Other philosophers take different views. In practical terms, the boundaries of negative liberty in any given country will be determined by its political and judicial institutions.

Positive liberty, on the other hand, refers to a person's 'freedom to' take ownership of their decisions and to realise their valued goals. It is the ability to pursue a life of one's own choosing and to act as one's own master. But, realising positive liberty often requires assistance or provision of opportunities by others or by the state, such as access to education, housing, or healthcare.[13] Such opportunities or assistance cannot be unrestricted, and will vary amongst different societies. As with negative liberty, the boundaries of positive liberty will be set by each nation's judicial and political institutions.

In a fair society, judicial and political institutions must weigh and balance individual liberties, both negative and positive, against public interests, that is, the interest of society as a whole. In the UK, senior judges have affirmed that, in case of medical treatment, negative liberty is absolute: as long as people have decision-making capacity, treatment cannot be imposed on them, regardless of the consequences of not doing so. Implicitly, judges have taken this approach to negative liberty because:

> We have too often seen freedom disappear in other countries not only by coups d'état but by gradual erosion: and often it is the first step that counts. So it would be unwise to make even minor concessions (pg. 43E).[14]

By contrast, positive liberty – a person's opportunities to access certain types of healthcare – is approached quite differently, as the next section will explore.

Prioritisation of public interest over self-determination in requesting treatment

The House of Lords has made it clear that the general principle of respect for autonomy does not extend to unqualified claims to receive treatment:

> Although the general rule is that the individual is the master of his own fate the judges through the common law have, in the public interest, imposed certain constraints on the harm that people may consent to being inflicted on their own bodies (pg. 70D).[15]

The Court of Appeal reinforced this point:

> Autonomy and the right of self-determination do not entitle the patient to insist on receiving a particular medical treatment regardless of the nature of the treatment. In so far as the doctor has a legal obligation to provide treatment this cannot be founded simply upon the fact that the patient demands it. The source of the duty lies elsewhere (para 31).[16]

The Court of Appeal did not specify this 'source of the duty': what is the justification that identifies treatments that a doctor is obliged to provide? The answer returns to the public interest. The 'source' of the doctor's duty lies in the public interest: only those types of treatment (and indications for such treatments) that are considered to be in the public interest will be regarded as reasonable treatments that doctors are obliged to make available to their patients.[17] Thus, public interest supplies justification for both withholding certain treatments and for making it legitimate to supply other treatments.

Now, if that the *End of Life Bill* is enacted, it will effectively declare that medical assistance in dying, subject to its provisions, aligns with the public interest. It is this public interest justification that would exempt doctors from the criminal law; and not simply the fact that a terminally ill patient requested, or consented to, assisted dying. Rather, it is because Parliament would have recognised such assistance as falling within the scope of lawful medical practice. Consent is only valid in law when the underlying treatment is lawful.[18,19]

An important question that now arises is whether assisted dying can be regarded as a 'medical treatment'. This is addressed in the next section.

Is assisted dying a medical treatment?

It can be debated whether assisted dying constitutes a 'proper medical treatment', or whether it belong to a novel and separate category of medical activity. The British Medical Association (BMA) has argued that assisted dying is not a 'treatment option' in the conventional sense.[20] Consequently (so the BMA's argument proceeds), existing laws pertaining to doctors' duties in providing treatment does not apply to assisted dying.

The opposing stance in this debate is that if assisted dying is recognised as a lawful and publicly justified intervention, it should be considered part of the range of treatment options for terminally ill patients. From this perspective, the Bill would broaden the spectrum of available care to include assisted dying as a legitimate medical service.

The Bill itself appears to support the BMA's more cautious stance. It adopts an 'opt-in' model: only doctors who voluntarily choose to participate are required to do so. Unlike a conscientious objection clause (such as that in the Abortion Act 1967), this opt-in model does not require a doctor to declare or explain their non-participation. This suggests that assisted dying is not being treated like a standard medical treatment, for which 'opt-out' is the exception.

That said, the legal status of assisted dying may ultimately be clarified only through case law, once the Act is implemented. In the meantime, doctors should be mindful of the ethical tensions embedded in both interpretations of assisted dying's status.

The legal principles of shared decision-making for a medical treatment

If assisted dying is held to be a conventional treatment option, then doctors' legal obligations regarding discussion and disclosure of assisted dying would follow the established framework of shared decision-making (SDM). As pointed out by the BMA, these obligations would be determined by the laws that have been set out by the Supreme Court in the cases of *Montgomery v Lanarkshire Health Board*[21] and *McCulloch v Forth Valley Health Board*.[22]

The *Montgomery-McCulloch* case pair sets out a two-stage model for SDM.[23] First, the doctor has to identify treatment options that are reasonable for each patient in the context of her or his individual situation (*McCulloch*).[24] Then, the doctor must discuss the material information about these options so that the patient can make an informed choice (*Montgomery*).[18,19]

Even with the legal protections that are provided by the Bill, the well-established and widely followed principles of SDM may pose ethical dilemma both for doctors who choose not to participate in assisted dying and for those who do opt in.

Ethical dilemmas for non-participating doctors

If assisted dying is not regarded as a medical treatment, are doctors still expected to inform patients of its availability under the Bill? Even if the doctor had not opted in, would the doctor bear the responsibility for, at least, making terminally ill patients aware that assisted dying was an option that was available to them?

The Bill makes is clear on this point. It states: 'no registered medical practitioner is under any duty to raise the subject of the provision of assistance' with the patient.[4] Instead, it is up to patient to express 'their wish to seek assistance to end their own life in accordance with this Act'; whereupon, doctors may undertake the preliminary assessment themselves or refer the patient to another doctor who is willing and able to do so. The Bill allows doctors to exercise their 'professional judgement to decide if, and when, it is appropriate to discuss the matter with a person'. But, the doctor is not obliged to do so.

The delegation of the initiative for discussing assisted dying to the patient conflicts with current legal expectations of SDM. For terminally ill patients to initiate the discussion, they must, at a minimum, know about the Bill and be sufficiently assertive and articulate to make the request for assistance in dying. This reverts to a discredited stance in consent law, where doctors were under no duty to disclose information unless specifically asked. As pointed out in *Montgomery*: 'there is something unreal about placing the onus of asking upon a patient who may not know that there is anything to ask about. It is indeed a reversal of logic' (para 58).[21]

Leaving the initiative to patients may disproportionately disadvantage those who are less informed, less articulate, or more vulnerable, thereby deepening health inequalities. While the BMA has proposed a separate 'assisted dying service', the Bill makes no explicit provision for such a service. Given that most terminally ill patients are under medical care and depend on their doctors for guidance, omitting any mention of assisted dying may create significant tensions in SDM.

Ethical dilemma for doctors who do 'opt in' to provide assisted dying

Doctors who opt in to provide assisted dying will play a vital role in advancing the terminally ill patient's request. Once a person makes a request to be provided with assistance to end their own life ('first declaration'), then at least two doctors (a co-ordinating doctor and an independent doctor) have to be satisfied that the person fulfils the provisions of the Bill, in order for the person's declaration to progress to the Assisted Dying Review Panel.

Besides determining objective criteria such as age and place of residence, the doctors are required to assess whether the person is terminally ill, has capacity to make the decision to end their own life and 'has a clear, settled and informed wish to end their own life'.[4] These assessments necessarily involve the exercise of medical professional judgments, commonly known as clinically judgments, that can be ethically challenging and contentious.

The nature of a clinical judgment - what exactly does it mean? is ill-defined. Broadly, there are two opposing points of view. On one view, a clinical judgment should be confined to technical issues only, such as scientific interpretation of data and application of evidence-based practice. An opposing view is that clinical judgments include a caring, emotional investment in the patient's wellbeing, such that the judgment includes a moral calculus: not only what can be done for the patient but also what ought to be done. In the first view, the patient's choice is seen as the primary moral consideration and the doctor's role is limited to issues of medical science. Whereas, the second view is relational: doctors see their role as that of a guide or philosopher who engages in a dialogue with patients and helps them to make wise choices.[25]

Contemporary ethical and legal emphasis on respect for patient autonomy would seem to support the technical view, where the doctor acts as a neutral facilitator. However, a nuanced analysis of respect for autonomy would argue that this ethical principle goes far beyond facilitating mere choice. Rather, it includes helping patients to navigate complex, value-laden decisions.[26] Indeed, the ethic of care that is widely endorsed in healthcare professions would support the latter view.

A recent study of doctors participating in medical assistance in dying (MAiD) in Canada captures the problem.[27] Some saw their role simply a 'conduit' for assisted dying, with moral (interpreted not as religion, but a wider view of what ought to be done) decision-making being left to the patients. Others conceived their role as 'conductors', who saw themselves as responsible for maintaining wider patient interests and preserving their own moral and professional integrity. A third group expressed ambivalence between these roles of conduit versus conductor.

The Canadian role distinctions in MAiD expose the spectrum of ethical responses and dilemmas that are likely to emerge in any jurisdiction where assisted dying is legalised, including the UK.

Conclusion

The legalisation of assisted dying, if realised, would represent a landmark shift in the relationship between law, medicine, and society in the UK. As discussed in this chapter, the *Terminally Ill Adults (End of Life) Bill* engages deeply with core tenets of medical jurisprudence, most notably the interplay between self-determination, public interest, and the nature of lawful medical treatment. It reveals how, in the UK's common law tradition, consent alone is insufficient to justify medical interventions unless they fall within the realm of treatments that are deemed to serve the public good.

Through an exploration of legal precedent and philosophical frameworks, such as Berlin's concepts of liberty, the chapter has highlighted the conceptual tensions that make assisted dying a unique ethical and legal challenge. Whether or not assisted dying is ultimately classified as a medical treatment, and regardless of a physician's choice to participate, clinicians must be equipped to navigate the emerging legal landscape with clarity and responsibility.

Ultimately, assisted dying is not solely a matter of individual choice or professional conscience. It is a legal institution grounded in societal values, requiring rigorous professional judgment, sensitive communication, and ethical integrity. The path forward demands a nuanced understanding of the law: not merely to comply with it, but to honour the values it seeks to uphold.

References

1. Gostin LO, Monahan JT, Kaldor J, et al. The legal determinants of health: harnessing the power of law for global health and sustainable development. Lancet. 2019;393:1857–1910.

2. Sarela AI. Can medical ethics truly be independent of law? J Med Ethics. 2024;50:177–178.

3. Huxtable R. Safeguarding assisted dying—court or committee? BMJ. 2025;388:r440.

4. Terminally Ill Adults (End of Life) Bill, 2025.

5. *Airedale NHS Trust v Bland* [1993] AC 789 (HL).

6. Lewis P. The medical exception. Curr Leg Probl. 2012;65(1):355–376.

7. *Re T (Adult: Refusal of Treatment)* [1993] Fam 95 (CA).

8. *Aintree University Hospitals NHS Foundation Trust v James* [2013] UKSC 67, [2014] AC 591.

9. Bagehot. Assisted dying and the two concepts of liberty. Economist. 20 November 2024.

10. Berlin I. Two concepts of liberty. Oxford University Press, 1969.

11. Rawls J. Justice as fairness. A restatement. Kelly E, ed. Harvard University Press, 2001.

12. Mill JS. On liberty and other writings. Collini S, ed. first published 1859. Cambridge University Press, 1989.

13. Sen A. The idea of justice. Penguin Books, 2010.

14. *S (An Infant) v S* [1972] AC 24 (HL).

15. *Re F (Mental Patient: Sterilisation)* [1990] 2 AC 1 (HL).

16. *R (on the application of Burke) v General Medical Council* [2005] EWCA Civ 1003, [2006] QB 273.

17. Sarela AI. Consent: what are 'reasonable' and 'available' treatments? Bull Roy Coll Surgeons Engl. 2024;106(4). Published online only.

18. Sarela AI. Consent for medical treatment: what is 'reasonable'? Health Care Anal. 2023;32:47–62.

19. Sarela AI. Does the General Medical Council's 2020 guidance on consent advance on its 2008 guidance? J Med Ethics. 2022;48:948–951.

20. Association BM. Physician assisted dying. Available from: https://www.bma.org.uk/advice-and-support/ethics/end-of-life/physician-assisted-dying.

21. *Montgomery v Lanarkshire Health Board* [2015] UKSC 11, [2015] AC 1430.

22. *McCulloch and others v Forth Valley Health Board* [2023] UKSC 26, [2023] 3 WLR 321.

23. Sarela AI, Miola J, Oliver K, Badenoch J, Selby P. Legal principles of shared decision-making for healthcare: what are we required to do? J R Soc Med. 2025;118:109–111.

24. Sarela AI. The Supreme Court's decision in *McCulloch v Forth Valley Health Board*: Does it condone healthcare injustice? J Med Ethics. 2024;50:806–810.

25. Sarela AI. Basma v Manchester University Hospitals NHS Foundation Trust: the scrutiny of a clinical judgement. Med Law Rev. 2021;29:728–739.

26. Sarela AI. Using legal doctrine and feminist theory to move beyond shared decision making for the practice of consent. Clin Ethics. 2023;18:361–367.

27. Winters JP, Walker S, Pickering NJ, Jaye C. Conduit or conductor? Physician providers' descriptions of their role as MAiD assessors in the first years after legalisation in Canada. J Med Ethics. 2025: Published Online First: 07 May 2025. doi: 10.1136/jme-2024-110518. Online ahead of print.PMID: 40335281

Chapter 11: Discussion

The principal purpose of our workshop and book in 2020[1] and of this update is to provide and review the international experience with AD to inform debate and process. In the workshop and subsequent publication, there was a consensus that the decisions about changing legislation should be influenced most by social, legal and political opinion and should not be heavily influenced by those of healthcare professionals. In this updated version we expand and refresh the international experience of AD and seek to inform readers of the current situation around the world and perspectives and evidence from a range of viewpoints and opinions.

The knowledge and views of healthcare professionals are important, not primarily because they should guide or shape public opinion but because these professionals are closely involved in the provision of good-quality care for patients at the end of life and will continue to be so. Any legislative change will have a very substantial impact on the patterns and quality of clinical practice and communication with patients.

The UK Chief Medical Officers have clearly advised "*This has to be a decision for society as a whole, expressed through Parliament*".[2] It now seems likely that UK (England/Wales and Scotland) and other British Isles, legislation will be enacted in the reasonably near future. Healthcare professionals must play a major role in its refinement and the meticulous planning for its implementation.

The arguments between supporters and opponents of AD are often strongly felt and often divisive. It is difficult to gain an overview of their nature. Box and Chambaere analysed the reported content of eight parliamentary debates[3] and summarised the "poles" of opinion. Those in support of AD legislation emphasised autonomy and compassion and described examples of deaths with poor control of suffering. Opponents argued that disadvantaged people would suffer inappropriate pressure to access AD, that healthcare systems would have to bear costs that would damage other services, and that, even if the legislation was to permit AD only for "terminal illness with an estimated life expectancy", as in the current Bill before Westminster, then there would be a pressure to extend the criteria to "intolerable suffering". Cultural and religious issues and evidence were mentioned but were relatively uncommon.

Public opinion about AD has been studied for decades and there are stable indications of a majority in favour of making AD for "Terminal Illness with an estimated life expectancy" legal in a wide variety of surveys, including those which describe closely the details of what is proposed, and about which questions are posed. This is less clear for AD when eligibility extends to those with "Intolerable Suffering without a terminal diagnosis or an estimated life expectancy".

The international experience is divided into two different approaches to eligibility for AD. While all jurisdictions require that the person who requests AD must be mentally competent, have a settled intent and be free to choose, they differ in the key eligibility requirements between

- "Terminal illness". In this case the person must have a diagnosis which is causing suffering, and which is reasonably expected to lead to their deaths within a defined timeframe, commonly 6 months or 12 months.
- "Intolerable suffering". In this case, no defined timeframe is required.

In jurisdictions where both are permitted, most AD cases are in the Terminal Illness "track", such as over 90% currently in Canada.

These two very different sets of eligibility criteria, present different requirements and influence the provision of the service. Jurisdictions which use the Terminal illness eligibility (the majority) have lower proportions of people receiving AD as a proportion of total deaths, than those using the "Intolerable suffering" criterion.

There are also two broadly different approaches to the administration of the medicines in AD

- Self-administration
- Administration by a healthcare professional

Some jurisdictions permit both. Jurisdictions which permit only self-administration have lower proportions of people receiving AD than those that permit administration by a healthcare professional.

Current proposals for the UK (England and Wales, Scotland) and British Isles are for a Terminal Illness eligibility requirement and self-administration of medication.

There is now a substantial body of international experience which we have reviewed in this publication which demonstrates that it is possible to legally permit AD and to deliver appropriate services safely, if a society and its legislators so decide. The recent experience in New Zealand and Australia is particularly relevant to the UK because the eligibility for AD which has been established in their law, is very similar to that proposed in the UK and British Isles. The experience in those countries is described in government reports and academic papers and brought together in preceding chapters. Compliance with regulation is closely monitored and procedures to improve the delivery of the AD services as experience accrues, is in place.

The longer experience in the USA is also relevant to the UK/British Isles because the eligibility criteria and methods to deliver AD are similar to those proposed in the UK/British Isles. However, US healthcare systems are very different to those in the UK and direct comparisons are more difficult.

Canadian experience has a great deal to teach us, and it shows that AD can be safely delivered but with the complex challenges we described in Chapter 5. We noted the quite rapid progression of eligibility criteria driven by court rulings, and the uncertainties around some eligibility criteria for MAiD, such as mental illness. The outcomes of the proposed current changes in Canada will be carefully followed in other jurisdictions. The need for a proactive approach to regulation and training to promote a consistent patient experience across a large federal country, is well illustrated in Canada.

European experience of AD divides into two. First, long term and stable delivery of AD in the Benelux countries provides valuable data but the eligibility criteria are very different from those in the USA, New Zealand and Australia and those proposed for the UK. Second, the emerging experience in other European countries is probably too early to provide robust insights. We noted the close integration of AD into Palliative Care in Austria, and it will be important to follow that experience.

There are many ethical and practical challenges. Many healthcare professionals are at the forefront of delivering changes internationally. The evidence suggests that this can generate challenging experiences ethically for some and that many find the processes and procedures of AD difficult and demanding. This may remain the case even in countries with long term experience of AD and for most of them this is an uncomfortable and uncertain experience, especially at the outset. This needs to be recognised. The healthcare professionals involved are facing a substantial change from the expectations upon which they were trained and steep "learning curves". There is some evidence particularly from North America that specialisation in AD is emerging from several medical disciplines and from nursing.

Healthcare professionals recognise, without exceptions, that the most important healthcare service for patients with terminal disease is accessible and adequately resourced Palliative Care. However, international experience shows that even when Palliative Care is provided, a small proportion of patients still choose AD. The proportion of people who choose AD is in the order of 2% of all deaths currently internationally, and it depends critically on their diagnosis with the large majority having a diagnosis of cancer or neurodegenerative diseases.

There is a universal international approach to the essential safeguards to ensure that requests for AD are freely made, conform to the eligibility requirements and that vulnerable people are protected. The conclusion in 2020 that *"The evidence from these jurisdictions suggests that the legal criteria that apply to an individual's request for AD are well respected: individuals who receive AD do so on the basis of valid requests; third parties who assist individuals to die do not act unlawfully"*,[2] remains the case. We are unaware of evidence that the situation is changed. However, there can be no place for complacency and rigorous scrutiny, reporting and monitoring is required in all the newer permissive jurisdictions.

Healthcare professionals have serious concerns about the delivery of AD to protect their patients and to ensure the quality and capacity of the care service is adequate. Ethical and religious concerns are expressed but, more commonly, it is the practical and professional issues that dominate the literature. Training, specialisation, sufficient time, numbers of trained staff, protection of personal beliefs and professional standing are all prominent concerns. Robust properly resourced clinical and support services are essential.

Neurodegenerative diseases present a distinct challenge to planning services for AD and several jurisdictions have identified special provisions for them, to take account, if possible, of the tempo of these diseases and their risk of loss of mental or physical capacity. These diseases are central to the planning of legislation and the implementation of new laws

The international peer reviewed literature on patient and caregiver experience of AD shows that it must be meticulously planned at both patient centred and technical levels. The reports on patient and caregiver experiences are broadly reassuring but examples of complications and unsettling experiences do occur uncommonly. The existence of the international experience must be a major asset to ensure that the UK service, which may be going to be undertaking this work at a challenging time, should be able to benefit from that experience and get things close to right, and monitor and improve them thereafter.

Cultural and religious beliefs and the views of disadvantaged and/or disabled people are a vitally important part of the debates about AD and have to be considered in the implementations and monitoring of any legislation changes. They are complex issues and there is not always a consensus among the groups. The international literature shows that, in general, people and organisations with strong religious views are more likely to be opposed to AD than those without these beliefs and they must be afforded the right to follow their consciences. The views of disabled and/ or vulnerable people were discussed in detail in Chapter 8 and there does not seem to be a consensus about changes in the law to permit AD. However, their views must be considered and if the law changes, they should have input into monitoring procedures.

UK healthcare practice, especially in Oncology, is built around multidisciplinary/multiprofessional team working, with good evidence that there are measurable benefits to patients from this approach.[4] The challenges presented by implementing an accessible, high quality, person-centred and safe service for AD are most likely to be met by a similar approach. Internationally, General practitioners and oncologists make up the majority of medical practitioners involved in AD internationally. Adequate resources and capacity for AD services will be essential. However, experience in oncology shows us that patients will need multidisciplinary care with input and support of many healthcare professionals especially nurses.

Palliative care professionals' input into the ultimate delivery of the service may well be numerically quite small as in other countries, but their role will be essential to ensure that the patient and the whole team are fully informed about palliative care options at all stages of their illness. Oncologists whether Clinical, Medical or Surgical must provide information about the active treatment options for patients and are best placed to provide the most accurate estimates of a patient prognosis and the point at which it is reasonable to say that, on the balance of probabilities they have a reasonable chance of dying within 6 months. The integration of such a multiprofessional approach require excellence in the administrative support and the information systems that are used.

International experience is a vital resource to guide us in decision and detail in the UK in the coming discussions and decisions. As a society and for those in decision making positions, whether legislative or medical, the experience and evidence from others should aid development of any AD service should it be legalised and we should take care to note, respect and consider all opinions, reflections and guidance in this sphere.

References

1. Board R, Bennett MI, Lewis P, Wagstaff J, Selby P, eds. End of life choices for cancer patients. An international perspective. Oxford: EBN Health, 2020.

2. UK chief medical officers and NHS England National Medical Director, 2024. Assisted Dying debate: advice to doctors. https://www.gov.uk/government/publications/assisted-dying-bill-debate-advice-to-doctors

3. Box G, Chambaere K. The use of arguments and justifications in Westminster parliamentary debates on assisted dying. Health Policy. 2024;144:105059.

4. Velikova G, Fallowfield L, Younger J, Board R, Selby P, eds. Problem solving in patient-centred and integrated cancer care. Oxford: EBN Health, 2018.

Chapter 12: Voluntary Assisted Dying – Plain Language Summary

The aim of this update is to give a clear, balanced overview of international experience with Voluntary Assisted Dying (VAD), principally to inform the ongoing debates in the UK/British Isles and other jurisdictions. It draws on the published medical literature especially where a topic has been systematically reviewed to include as much of the literature as possible. It also includes government reports, and official data from around the world to help inform public discussion. It updates our publication End of Life Choices for Cancer Patients (EBN Health) from 2020.

What Is Voluntary Assisted Dying (VAD)?

Different countries use different terms, but they generally mean similar things:

- *Assisted Dying* includes both euthanasia and assisted suicide.
- *Euthanasia* means a medical intervention intended to end a person's life to relieve suffering.
- *Assisted suicide* means giving someone the means to end their own life.
- *Physician-assisted death, Physician Assisted Suicide and Medical Assistance in Dying (MAiD)* are terms used in different countries, that may include both approaches.

Where It Is Legal

Laws allowing VAD exist in:

- *Europe:* The Netherlands, Belgium, Luxembourg, Spain, Portugal, Austria, and Switzerland.
- *North America:* Canada and some U.S. states (Washington, Oregon, Hawaii, California, Colorado, New Mexico, Maine, Vermont, New Jersey, and the District of Columbia).
- *Australasia:* All six Australian states and New Zealand.
- *Other countries:* Colombia, Germany, Italy, and Montana (USA) have partial permissions.

Together, in 2023, these countries represent about 282 million people. In the most recently reported time periods, about 2% of all deaths in these countries involved VAD, ranging from less than 1% to about 5% of all deaths — lowest in U.S. States and highest in Canada and the Netherlands.

Around three-quarters of VAD cases involve people with cancer or motor neurone disease and the other related conditions, which are referred to as neurodegenerative diseases, compared to around 30% of all deaths.

Rates are lower where only assisted suicide (not euthanasia) is allowed, or where patients must have a specific life expectancy (e.g., 6 or 12 months).

How Laws Differ

There are two main types of eligibility criteria:

1. *Terminal illness:* The person is dying from a disease expected to cause death within a defined period (usually 6–12 months).

2. *Intolerable suffering:* The person has severe suffering that cannot be relieved, without a set time-frame for death.

All jurisdictions require that people requesting VAD must:

- Be mentally competent,
- Make the decision freely and consistently, and
- Understand the consequences.

Where the law focuses on terminal illness, VAD usually accounts for a smaller proportion of all deaths. Countries which include "intolerable suffering" as a criterion for VAD (like Belgium and the Netherlands) have higher rates.

How It Works

Two main methods are used:

- *Self-administration:* The person takes the prescribed medicine themselves.
- *Clinician administration:* A healthcare professional gives the medicine.

Some countries permit both. Where only self-administration is allowed, fewer people use VAD.

Current UK Situation

In the UK and British Isles all forms of VAD are currently illegal. However, in England and Wales, Scotland, Jersey, and the Isle of Man changes in legislation are being discussed in their Parliaments. Proposals generally include:

- *Terminal illness* as the eligibility requirement
- *Self-administration* of medication

Each jurisdiction is at a different stage, but all have seen growing parliamentary support for change.

In our workshop and subsequent 2020 publication, there was a consensus that the decisions about changing legislation should be influenced most by social, legal and political opinions and should not be heavily influenced by those of healthcare professionals. The knowledge and views of healthcare professionals are important, not primarily because they should guide or shape public opinion but because these professionals are closely involved in the provision of good-quality care for patients at the end of life and will continue to be so. Any legislative change will have a very substantial impact on the patterns and quality of clinical practice and communication with patients. The UK Chief Medical Officers have clearly advised *"This has to be a decision for society as a whole, expressed through Parliament"*.

It now seems likely that in the UK (England/Wales and Scotland) and other British Isles, legislation will be enacted in the reasonably near future. Healthcare professionals must play a major role in its refinement and the meticulous planning for its implementation.

The arguments between supporters and opponents of VAD are often strongly felt and often divisive. In UK parliamentary debates, those in support of VAD legislation changes emphasised autonomy and compassion and described examples of deaths with poor control of suffering. Opponents argued that disabled or disadvantaged people would suffer inappropriate pressure to access AD, that healthcare systems would have to bear costs that would damage other services, and that, even if the legislation was to permit AD only for "terminal illness", as in the current Bill before Westminster, then there would be a pressure to extend the criteria to "intolerable suffering".

International Experience and Lessons

There is now a substantial body of international experience, which we have reviewed in this publication, which demonstrates that it is possible to legally permit VAD and to deliver appropriate services safely with strong oversight and training, if a society and its legislators so decide. The recent experience in New Zealand and Australia is particularly relevant to the UK, because the eligibility for VAD, which has been established in their law is very similar to that proposed in the UK and British Isles. The international experience is described in government reports and academic papers and brought together in preceding chapters. Compliance with regulation is closely monitored and procedures to improve the delivery of the VAD services, as experience accrues, are in place.

- *New Zealand and Australia* have models similar to what is proposed in the UK, with strict regulation and continuous review.
- *Ten of the United States* have long experience under "death with dignity" laws. Although healthcare systems differ, compliance and reporting are closely monitored.
- *Canada's system* (MAiD) demonstrates both the benefits and challenges of wider access, including an ongoing intense debate about extending eligibility for VAD to people with mental illness.
- *Benelux countries (Belgium, Netherlands, Luxembourg)* have had VAD for over 20 years and report stable systems, though eligibility is broader than in other regions.

Across all jurisdictions, strong regulation and professional training are essential.

Ethical and Professional Challenges

Assisted dying raises difficult moral and emotional issues for healthcare staff. The medical literature in all of the countries, even those with decades of experience, still contains reports that healthcare professionals can find involvement with VAD difficult and challenging. Some now specialise in VAD to manage the ethical and technical complexities.

All agree that high-quality palliative care remains essential and is a vital service to be provided for many patients with serious illnesses, including those who are reaching the end of their lives. Adequate resources for palliative care are essential in all healthcare systems. Most patients who choose VAD have already received palliative care but want control over the timing, location and nature of their death.

International evidence supports the conclusion that when laws are properly designed and regulated:

- Requests are made voluntarily and lawfully
- Safeguards protect vulnerable people
- Compliance with legal requirements is high

However, continuous oversight and transparency remain crucial.

Cultural and Religious Views, Disabled People and Vulnerable Groups

Cultural and religious beliefs and the views of disadvantaged and/or disabled people are a vitally important part of the debates about AD and have to be considered in the implementation and monitoring of any legislation changes. They are complex issues and there is not always a consensus among the groups.

Views among disabled people are divided. Some fear that VAD could make them feel less valued or pressured. Others see it as a way to maintain autonomy if they face a terminal illness.

So far, data do not show that disabled people are overrepresented among those choosing VAD, but long-term monitoring and involvement of disabled groups in oversight are essential.

Cultural and religious beliefs strongly shape opinions. Most religious organisations oppose VAD, while public support is higher among those without religious affiliation.

Public Opinion in the UK

Surveys over many years show consistent majority support in the UK for allowing VAD in cases of terminal illness with limited life expectancy. Support is weaker for allowing it in cases of intolerable suffering without terminal illness.

In countries where both options exist, most VAD cases (e.g., 90% in Canada) are for terminal illness.

What Healthcare Systems Need

Introducing VAD requires:

- Well-trained, multidisciplinary teams
- Clear administrative and IT systems
- Interaction with palliative care services
- Strong professional support and ethical guidance

Doctors, nurses, and allied professionals must have access to training, supervision, and the ability to opt out on grounds of conscience. The introduction of VAD into a healthcare system is a huge challenge to healthcare professionals, changing many aspects of their work and communications with seriously ill patients.

Many healthcare professionals are concerned about the introduction of VAD because the system is under great pressure at the moment. The provision of VAD must be adequately resourced and carefully planned. Waiting lists and cancellations would be unacceptable where access and the timeliness of VAD was affected.

Neurodegenerative diseases, such as motor neurone disease, need special planning because of the risk of losing mental or physical capacity before a decision can be acted on.

Conclusion

More than 280 million people live in countries where some form of assisted dying is legal. International evidence shows that with clear rules, strong safeguards, and professional support, VAD can be provided safely and respectfully.

If, in the UK and British Isles, we decide to change the law, it can learn from decades of international experience — especially from Australia and New Zealand over the last 5 years — to design a system that protects vulnerable people, supports healthcare professionals, and respects individual choice.